JOHN MARTYN CHAMBERLAIN

MEDICAL REGULATION, FITNESS TO PRACTISE AND REVALIDATION

A Critical Introduction

POLICY PRESS SHORTS RESEARCH

First published in Great Britain in 2015 by

Policy Press
University of Bristol
1-9 Old Park Hill
Bristol
BS2 8BB
UK
t: +44 (0)117 954 5940
pp-info@bristol.ac.uk
www.policypress.co.uk

North America office:
Policy Press
c/o The University of Chicago Press
1427 East 60th Street
Chicago, IL 60637, USA
t: +1 773 702 7700
f: +1 773 702 9756
sales@press.uchicago.edu
www.press.uchicago.edu

British Library Cataloguing in Publication Data
A catalogue record for this book is available from the British Library.

Library of Congress Cataloging-in-Publication Data
A catalog record for this book has been requested.

ISBN 978-1-4473-2544-4 (hardcover)
ISBN 978-1-4473-2546-8 (ePub)
ISBN 978-1-4473-2547-5 (Mobi)

Cover design by Andrew Corbett
Front cover: image kindly supplied by Getty
Printed and bound in Great Britain by CMP, Poole
Policy Press uses environmentally responsible print partners

For Jane and Freyja

Contents

List of tables   vi
About the author   vii

1   Governing medicine: from gentlemen's club to risk-based regulation   1

2   Fitness to practise in the workplace: medical revalidation   23

3   Fitness to practise panels: the Medical Practitioners Tribunal Service   59

4   Regulating for the safer doctor in the risk society: is the process the punishment?   79

Notes   97
Appendix   *The Good Medical Practice Framework for Appraisal and Revalidation*   99
Index   105

List of tables

1	Number of complaints received by the GMC (1995–2012)	67
2	Source of enquiry (1995-2012)	68
3	Enquiries received and concluded (2006-2012)	69
4	Breakdown of GMC investigatory action outcomes (2006-2012)	70
5	Fitness to practise panel outcomes	71

About the author

Dr John Martyn Chamberlain is associate professor in medical criminology at the University of Southampton. His academic background covers criminology, medical sociology and socio-legal studies. His primary research interests include the study of medical malpractice, negligence and criminality, as well as the role played by specialist forms of medical and healthcare expertise in the identification and governance of 'troublesome' social groups, including people who are unwell, 'deviant' and criminally insane. Drawing on this background, he has written widely on medical-legal developments in the regulation and discipline of doctors, including the book *Doctoring Medical Governance: Medical Regulation in Transition*, which was runner-up for the 2010 British Sociological Association sociology of health and illness book of the year.

Second

GOVERNING MEDICINE: FROM GENTLEMEN'S CLUB TO RISK-BASED REGULATION

Introduction

Over the last two decades there has been heightened political, legal and public interest in the field of doctors' fitness to practise as a result of a series of medical regulatory failings in prominent medical malpractice cases, such as the respective Bristol and Alder Hey cases, as well as medical acts of criminality, including multiple homicide in the case of the general practitioner Harold Shipman (Chamberlain, 2012). Consequently, the question of how best to legislate to protect those in need of medical treatment from the incompetent and criminal actions of doctors is of fundamental significance and interest to members of the public, government, practitioners, academics and lawyers, among others.

This book examines the topic of medical fitness to practise and revalidation, and how we as a society ensure that doctors remain competent in their chosen specialty through a critical sociolegal lens that draws on the disciplinary fields of medical sociology, criminology and law. Revalidation involves a thorough assessment of a doctor's fitness to practise using a mixture of appraisals, patient feedback and continuing professional development activities. It is the first time that doctors have been required by law to submit themselves to a regular performance appraisal of their practice, if they wish to stay on the medical register and continue to legally practise medicine in the United Kingdom (UK) [1].

First introduced in 2012, but not being completely rolled out nationally until 2016, and still very much being implemented for the first time at the time of writing, revalidation has been positioned by government and medical elites as being a new transparent and inclusive regulatory tool designed to modernise medical governance as well as to better ensure patient safety and health service delivery. Furthermore, in regard to the hearing of complaints against a doctor via medical fitness to practise panels (FPPs), the General Medical Council (GMC) has sought to address concerns regarding possible institutional bias by establishing the Medical Practitioners Tribunal Service (MPTS) in 2012 (GMC 2013). While in 2014 the Law Commission's comprehensive review of healthcare professionals noted that medical FPPs are a vitally important legal mechanism for ensuring that public trust in medical regulation is maintained when complaints are made about a doctor. Consequently it has acted to strengthen the investigatory and adjudication process, by legislating to ensure that they are autonomous structures, independent of the GMC (Law Commission 2014a, 2014b, 2014c).

As a result, this book is extremely timely and pertinent. It possesses a high level of public and academic interest, and it is hoped that its contents will generate a considerable degree of professional interest and practice-based impact. At its centre lies a concern with exploring on both practical and conceptual levels the consequences of two interlinked ideas: first, the idea that, as an occupation which possesses specialist expertise and a strong ethical 'service orientation', doctors can be left alone to manage their affairs, including the training, monitoring and disciplining of group members; and second, that once qualified, a doctor can be left alone to practise until they retire.

These two ideas have long defined the contractual nature of the relationship between profession and public under the legislative terms of the principle of self-regulation, as enshrined into law by the Medical Act 1858. But as the following chapters will explore, although they still do very much possess a degree of intellectual legitimacy and practical utility, under the conditions of the respective Health and Social Care Act 2008 and Health and Social Care Act 2012, they are now recognised (in legislative terms at least) as being well past their sell-by-date.

However, this does not mean that they have been completely eradicated from the professional and sociopolitical discourse surrounding how best to regulate medicine as a profession. Rather, as we shall see, they linger on, influencing the day-to-day practice of medicine and its quality assurance processes and practices. Indeed, this book is written for academics, practitioners, policy makers and regulatory and professional associations, precisely because how we as a society make sure our doctors are fit to practise is still very much a highly contested issue.

Before we explore the introduction of medical revalidation and FPP reforms in more detail, it is important to examine the changing regulatory and legal context through which it has emerged, and furthermore, to do so from a historical frame of reference based in the unfolding development from the 19th century onwards of the distinctive body of knowledge and practice that we now call modern medicine. It is here, as we shall see, that we first encounter the idea that as they are members of an occupation that possesses specialist expertise and a strong ethical 'service orientation', doctors can – and should – be left alone to manage their affairs. Yet interestingly, it was not the persuasiveness of this idea based on the emerging rationalistic and scientific nature of medical practice that resulted in it being enshrined in law. Nor was it the ethical claim made by the fledgling profession to place the patient interest first and foremost, although undoubtedly this did play a key role in persuading the public and political elites of the need to grant medicine control over its governing institutions. Rather, it was the prevailing socioeconomic and political context in the UK and its dependence on 'club governance' models of legislative regulation that set the sociolegal scene for the following one hundred and fifty years.

Overview of the book

The rest of this chapter explores this broader regulatory context, to provide a necessary historical introduction to the following chapters, which focus on medical fitness to practise and revalidation.

Chapter Two looks at revalidation in detail, outlining its introduction, key features, and current policy and practice surrounding its implementation. In doing so, the chapter unpacks several key issues pertinent to its future development which, it is argued, together reinforce the need to take steps to ensure that the interests of the public and doctors and their professional associations are balanced.

This leads on to Chapter Three, which explores current developments in FPPs. As already noted, when a formal complaint is made that calls into question a practitioner's fitness to practise, these are a vitally important legal mechanism for ensuring that public trust in medical regulation is maintained. The chapter examines how recent proposed Law Commission reforms may unintentionally serve, in particular types of cases, to undermine the principles of swift, proportionate and effective legal responses to ensure public protection.

Finally, Chapter Four brings these points together into a concluding summary, proposing several key action points for the future of medical revalidation and fitness to practise.

Regulating medicine: the Medical Act 1858

The Medical Act 1858 established the GMC as a public institution responsible for oversight of a single register of 'approved medical practitioners' – the medical register (Larson 1978). Under the Act, only individuals whose names are on the medical register are permitted to call themselves medical practitioners, and (since its establishment in 1948) work as doctors in the National Health Service (NHS). The GMC, therefore, represents the principal formal legal mechanism for medical regulation in the UK: maintaining a register of accredited and licensed doctors, establishing the standards of practice, and investigating complaints. In short, it is concerned with market 'entry' (licensure) and 'exit' (removing the 'bad apples') (Allsop and Saks 2002). Given the broad remit of its regulatory powers, the question of who controls the GMC is an important one.

The Medical Act 1858 conferred de facto control to the medical profession in determining entry into, and exit from, this legally underwritten register of state-approved medical practitioners, because all GMC members were drawn exclusively from medicine's elite professional associations, in particular the Royal Colleges (Stacey 1992). Indeed, of the initial 24 board members, nine were represented directly the Royal Colleges, 12 by the universities whose representatives were senior members of the Colleges, and the remaining three were nominated on the advice of the Privy Council. There was no space for general practitioners. This did not change until an amendment to the Act in 1886, which allowed the profession to elect by postal vote five doctors from the profession as a whole. It was not until 1926 that the Privy Council chose to include one layperson on the GMC board, although it would not be until after the enactment of the Medical Act 1983 that lay members would become a regular feature of the GMC board membership.

Due to the specialised nature of their expertise and their ethical claim to serve the needs of their clients first and foremost, professional organisations have historically played an important role in regulating entry conditions to the professions and in establishing standards of professional conduct. Medicine is no different in this regard. It is generally agreed that the development of a unified and autonomous scientific knowledge base has been essential to the professional status of medicine and the establishment of medical control of the GMC (Freidson 2001). The increasing emphasis, from the late 18th century onwards, on laboratory-based experiments twinned with hospital-based clinical practice, to seek cures for common human ailments and diseases, has led over the last three centuries to the development of highly specialised and esoteric forms of medical knowledge and technology. Yet medicine's altruistic principles and close association with science are not the only reasons why it was granted control of the GMC. The Medical Act 1858 and the GMC were both reflections of the essentially pre-democratic political structure in which they were founded. As Moran (2004, 94) notes: 'because government was the product of an era of oligarchy, deference and social elitism it was the government of clubs … [and] the government of doctors was patterned on the club system'.

Moran cites Marquand (1988: 178), who in his analysis of the ideology of the broader Victorian governing style, said that the: '[a]tmosphere of British government was that of a club, whose members trusted each other to observe the spirit of the club rules, the notion that the principles underlying the rules should be clearly defined and publicly proclaimed was profoundly alien'.

This 'club mentality' approach to medical regulation continued into the 20th century. The eminent medical sociologist Margaret Stacey, who was a lay member of the GMC in the late 1970s and early 1980s, noted that it still retained the ethos of being an exclusive 19th-century 'gentlemen's club': 'In 1858 the GMC was effectively a gentlemen's club. Its promise that the public could trust those it registered amounted to ensuring that there were no "bounders" in the medical fraternity [sic] who would do dastardly things such as no gentleman would do' (Stacey 1992: 204).

Bristol, Shipman and the Health and Social Care Act 2008

This laissez-faire and paternalistic 'gentlemen's club' approach to medical regulation was, however, subject to greater challenge from the early 1980s onwards, by both the public and the media, as a result of a growing number of high-profile medical malpractice scandals. One particularly important case from the 1990s was the medical cover-up of poor surgical performance at Bristol Royal Infirmary. The three doctors involved in the Bristol case were Mr James Wisheart, Mr Janardan Dhasmana and Mr John Roylance. Between 1990 and 1993 Mr Wisheart carried out a procedure to correct a heart defect known as an atrioventricular septal defect, on 15 patients, of whom 9 died. His mortality rate was over 60%, which is considerably higher than acceptable levels. Dr Dhasmana's mortality rate for this operation of 10% was far lower and within acceptable limits. However, his clinical competency was called into question when he performed a highly complex procedure called an 'arterial switch operation'. Out of 38 of Dr Dhasmana's patients, 20 died. The national success rate is between 80% and 90%.

Subsequently, the parents of the children who died launched a local support group that complained to the GMC. The GMC found Mr Wisheart and Mr Roylance guilty of serious professional misconduct and struck them off the medical register. However, Mr Dhasmana was not struck off the register, because he made the decision not to continue to perform further arterial switch operations when he realised that his mortality rate was high. The children's parents and the media subsequently called for a public inquiry. Frank Dobson, the then Secretary of State for Health, stated on the BBC television programme *Newsnight* that he took the view that all three doctors should have been removed from the medical register, and he subsequently instigated a public inquiry.

The GMC was widely regarded as being too slow to act to discipline the doctors involved and the public inquiry, chaired by Professor Ian Kennedy between 1998 and 2001, reported extensively on the broader failings within the management and clinical systems of the NHS to efficiently and effectively identify poor performance (Bristol Royal Infirmary Inquiry 2001). It heavily criticised the hierarchical medical 'club culture' evident in the Bristol heart unit and the GMC response to the complaints it received (Smith 1998).

After Bristol, it was recognised by professional elites that medical regulation must endeavour to become more open and transparent. Yet it was not strictly a medical malpractice case, but rather an instance of a doctor possessing criminal intent, which engendered fundamental change in the regulation of medical expertise (Gladstone 2000). Harold Shipman, a general practitioner from Hyde in Manchester, was able to use his position to murder 215 of his patients (Soothill and Wilson 2005). It was not until after his conviction that the GMC struck Shipman off the medical register and admitted that a decade earlier he had, in fact, come before its FPP for prescription abuse (Department of Health 2001). The resulting inquiry, led by Dame Janet Smith, played a pivotal role in reforming medical control of the GMC (Smith 2005). At the end her governmental review of the Shipman case, Smith concluded that:

> For the majority of GMC members, the old culture of protecting the interests of doctors lingers on ... it seems ... that one of the fundamental problems facing the GMC is the perception, shared by many doctors, that it is supposed to be 'representing' them. It is not, it is regulating them. ... In fact the medical profession has a very effective representative body in the BMA, it does not need – and should not have – two. (Smith 2005: 1176)

The content of the Health and Social Care Act 2008 in relation to the regulation of medicine was, in many ways, enacted as a direct result of Smith's 2005 report. The Smith Report introduced several key reforms in the legal regulation of doctors, which the 2008 Act legally codified. It legislated for reform in the constitution of the GMC, and as a consequence, the organisation is now composed of lay, professional and educational representatives with no professional majority. Appointment to the GMC is made through open competition via the Public Appointments Commission, against specific set criteria. In addition, the GMC has direct and explicit lines of accountability to Parliament, not the Privy Council. Finally, the 2008 Act legislated for the creation of an independent body with supervisory powers over the GMC (and other health and social care professional regulators) in the form of a super-regulator, the Council for Healthcare Regulatory Excellence (CHRE), which since 2012 has been called the Professional Standards Authority (PSA).

This super-regulator was tasked with reviewing how the GMC responds to complaints and fitness to practise cases. Changes were introduced to the management of fitness to practise cases, with adjudication being undertaken by an independent tribunal rather than by GMC committee, while the level of evidence required to meet the 'realistic prospect test' was reduced from the criminal to civil standard of proof. Medical 'revalidation' was introduced: revalidation involves a systematic five-yearly assessment of a doctor's fitness to practise using a combination of annual appraisals, patient feedback and continuing professional development activities (Donaldson 2008). Revalidation began to be implemented nationally in 2012, with every doctor in the UK being included in the revalidation process by 2016 (NHS Revalidation Support Team 2014). Revalidation transforms the GMC from an incident-led, reactive regulatory institution to a proactive overseer of a rolling programme of performance review.

The introduction of revalidation, together with changes in GMC membership, reforms in the handling of fitness to practise cases, alongside the introduction by the state of legal regulatory oversight in the form of the CHRE/PSA, could be said to signal the end of medical control of the GMC. It is arguable that the accumulation of regulatory failures across the domain of professional regulation has prompted a shift from 'front-line professional regulator' to 'regulated self-regulation' (Allsop and Saks 2002). Professional regulators have become accountable to 'meso-regulators', who in turn are accountable to political institutions (Kaye 2006). There might well be some truth in this assertion. It is certainly no longer the case that doctors' professional associations, such as the Royal Colleges and medical schools, directly control the GMC and therefore the professional standards that govern their practices. Nonetheless, collegial structures and practices do continue to be the primary means of formal and informal medical control of professional practice.

Furthermore, given the specialised nature of medical expertise, some form of professionally led medical regulation is both necessary and in the public interest. The introduction of revalidation, in particular, demonstrates that any attempts to reform 'the medical club' must acknowledge that in most cases peer review remains the primary mechanism by which satisfactory performance can be legitimately defined and judged (Cranberg et al 2008). Consequently, medical control of regulatory practice continues to operate both formally and informally at the level of everyday clinical practice. The medical regulatory system's reliance on peer review can perhaps most clearly be seen in relation to the handling of fitness to practise cases, as it is here that medical expertise and technical knowledge often act as the final arbiter when it comes to defining the grounds for reasonable legal case judgment (Chamberlain 2012).

Medical expertise and professional discretion

At its core, the discipline of medicine involves the identification and inculcation of a body of expert knowledge mastered through a period of prolonged education and training. Consequently, there is a logical consistency between the scientific foundations of modern medical expertise, the principle of medical self-regulation and the doctrine of clinical freedom. Given the specialised nature of medicine, patients typically prefer that doctors possess the freedom to decide the best course of treatment for them (clinical freedom), although it can be argued that the esoteric nature of medical knowledge infers that only a doctor's peers, rather than their patient, can be said to be sufficiently qualified to judge the quality of clinical work and if indeed the best course of treatment has been undertaken (medical self-regulation). For example, the Merrison Inquiry, which examined the regulation of medicine during the 1970s when the GMC first began to be subject to challenge, concluded:

> It is the essence of a professional skill that it deals with matters unfamiliar to the lay man, and it follows that only those in the profession are in a position to judge many of the matters of professional competence and conduct which will be involved. (Merrison 1975: 7)

The principle of medical self-regulation and clinical freedom is situated within legal precedent. To provide medical treatment, a doctor must exercise their discretion and make a clinical judgement regarding the best course of action to follow. Professional discretion requires doctors to assess and evaluate cases and conditions, and assert their professional judgement regarding advice, performance and treatment. Hence, underlying the notion of discretion is the concept of autonomy. Inextricably bound to the notion of autonomy is the notion of restriction, as there are always countervailing forces acting to constrain freedom. Dworkin's (1977: 31) description highlights the relative nature of the concept: 'discretion, like the hole in a doughnut, does not exist except for an area left open by a surrounding belt of restriction'.

Dworkin also distinguished between three different forms of discretion: weak, strong and official. Weak discretion refers to the need to exercise judgement when rules for action cannot simply be applied mechanistically, and is often found in large-scale bureaucratic organisations. Official discretion, itself a form of weak discretion, refers to a decision maker having the authority to make a final decision. Strong discretion, on the other hand, leaves both the decision making and the criteria of decision making to the individual. It is this type of discretion that is typically exerted by professionals operating in fields such as medicine and law (Jones 2011). Hence, to protect their strong discretionary freedom from 'outsiders' (other occupational groups and patients) who seek to restrain it, members of the medical profession close ranks and venerate the freedom of the individual practitioner and the existence of clinical judgement and expertise, although this is tempered by the presence of 'in-house' forms of informal and formal social control in relation to medical decision making when it goes awry (Evetts 2002).

Formal forms of collegiate control might include the traditional humiliation-by-teaching ward round for the medical trainee. More informal social control mechanisms are known to include the 'quiet chat' or use of 'protective support', where work is quietly shifted away from the 'problem doctor' (Irvine 2003). In examining the operation of informal social controls within medicine, Bosk (1978) distinguishes between technical and moral errors. Bosk posits that technical errors are treated less harshly than moral transgressions, because it is believed that the former can happen to anyone, but the latter are perceived as a rejection of shared social codes and values inculcated during medical training. He argues that while technical errors can be dealt with less conspicuously in most cases, moral errors demand public punishment to restore good faith in the profession as a whole. Formal mechanisms for responding to poor conduct by doctors operate at the local NHS Trust level via employment disciplinary proceedings as well as at the national level via the GMC. Furthermore, the emphasis placed on informal and formal 'in-house' social control and strong discretion within medicine in the face of countervailing forces seeking to monitor and curtail clinical autonomy, has a legal basis in medical negligence case law in the form of the *Bolam test*.[2]

The 'Bolam test' and the 'Bolitho gloss'

In cases of alleged clinical negligence, the minimum standard of care is determined by what is referred to as the *Bolam test*, following the McNair J direction in *Bolam v Friem Hospital Management Committee*.[3] According to the test, a defendant: 'is not guilty of negligence if he had acted in accordance with a practice accepted as proper by a responsible body of medical [persons] skilled in that particular art'.[4]

Under *Bolam*, therefore, the standard of care is set by the medical profession and evidenced by expert medical testimony, with minimal judicial scrutiny. In *Sadaxazy v Board of Governors of the Bethlem Royal Hospital and the Maudsley Hospital*, Scarman LCJ affirmed that 'the standard of care is a matter of medical judgement'.[5] Although there is case law support for the pre-eminence of peer review, just as medical self-regulation has been amended to include a regulatory oversight capable of questioning medical judgement, so has *Bolam*. Traditionally, courts tend not to take issue with clinical judgement that has been endorsed by expert testimony. However, in the last two decades they have increasingly examined the reasoning behind clinical decisions. This is known as the *Bolitho gloss*.[6] In *Bolitho v City and Hackney Health Authority*, Browne-Wilkinson LJ observed that:

> The court has to be satisfied that the exponents of the body of opinion relied upon can demonstrate that such opinion has a logical basis. In particular, in cases involving, as they so often do, the weighing of risks against benefits, the judge before accepting a body of opinion as being responsible, reasonable or respectable, will need to be satisfied that, in forming their views, the experts have directed their minds to the question of comparative risks and benefits and have reached a defensible conclusion on the matter.[7]

This suggests that the court should adopt a more interventionist stance in assessing expert evidence and in setting the standard of care. One approach towards a more objective measure in determining the legal standard of care is through the use of clinical guidelines. These are consensus statements, grounded in systematic evidence and designed to ensure the effectiveness and efficiency of medical care, to assist doctors in making decisions about treatment for specific conditions.

The *Bolitho gloss* reasserts the primacy of the court's role in scrutinising professional practice and expert witnesses, using tools such as clinical guidelines, for the purposes of the adversarial process (Samanta et al 2006). This highlights that medical discretion and expert opinion may be essential for the operation of regulatory regimes, but nevertheless they have increasingly become subject to non-medical third-party review, both in court and in the NHS.

The legislating measures undertaken to reform the GMC raise the question of their effects on outcomes: has the number of doctors removed from the medical register increased as a result of changes in the level of evidence needed to pass the 'realistic prospect test'? Chapter Three considers this question in more detail, outlining empirical data pertaining to FPP outcomes and critically evaluating proposed further reforms to the case investigation and hearing process. For the moment it is necessary to focus on the shift to risk-based regulation and the consequences of this for medical revalidation, in order to provide a necessary background for Chapter Two.

The shift to risk-based regulation

Dame Janet Smith, in her review of the GMC and its response to enquiries, concluded that the GMC was guilty of protecting the interests of doctors rather than patients. It has been observed in the context of the governance of the health and social welfare professions that increasing third-party questioning of medical expertise and entrenched professional interests is symbolic of the fact that we live in 'the age of risk-based regulation' (Hood and Miller 2010). It is this author's contention that the reforms outlined in this chapter provide supporting evidence for the argument that an organisational and cultural shift towards a risk-averse regulatory model has occurred as the GMC has been reformed in order to regain public trust in its decision-making processes (see, for example, GMC 2013).

The GMC, in its published reports, certainly advocates a risk-based model of regulation. Risk-based regulation relies heavily on seemingly objective decision-making processes, whereby codified forms of knowledge are used to prescribe performance targets and best-evidenced judgemental norms surrounding what constitutes appropriate action in a given situation (Lloyd-Bostock and Hutter 2008). This is concomitant with the regulatory shift from 'front-line professional regulator' to 'regulated self-regulation', which has occurred in the UK across the health and social care professions.

Rather than being a clearly defined method, risk-based regulation is best conceived of as a cluster of tools that provide rules for action and, in doing so, serve to constrain what action can be recorded in the first place. For example, a computer system called Siebel is used by the GMC to manage its complaint enquiry process:

> Siebel's pre-defined decision codes are expressed as the legal rule or section that has been applied. ... Where identification of risks is concerned, the coding of allegations is crucial. The allegation codes used in Siebel are designed, not to capture what is alleged, but rather to define a potential case within the GMC's powers. (Lloyd-Bostock 2010)

The use by the GMC of the Siebel computer system to support a relatively consistent administrative approach in responding to complaints, exemplifies a growing organisational reliance on codified, risk-averse, procedural rules to assist in the day-to-day processing of cases. As previously discussed, the outcomes of GMC activity are now subject to the 'meso-regulator' the PSA, and a key function of this additional layer of regulatory oversight is to promote a 'risk-averse' working culture of transparency and professional accountability. This is achieved through the proactive use of outcome data to establish clear performance standards and best-evidenced protocols and guidelines to inform decision-making processes in order to monitor organisational performance and ensure that regulatory standards are being maintained. In this context, it is clear why the use of Siebel is advocated, as it supports the development of a risk-based approach to regulation via the collection and sharing of outcome data to support institutional transformation.

The focus on risk-based regulation within the health and social care professions embodies a movement away from an incident-led, reactive regulatory approach (as traditionally exemplified by bodies such as the GMC), and towards proactive oversight of a rolling programme of performance review. In this context, patient complaint and FPP outcome data becomes one of medicine's new 'visible markers of trust [which as] … tools of bureaucratic regulation fulfil [a] function as signifiers of quality' (Kuhlmann 2006, 617). As such, they allow both the GMC and the PSA (which subjects it to regulatory oversight), to reaffirm the primacy of patient treatment and care in the face of previous high-profile instances of medical malpractice and criminality (Secretary of State for Health 2007). Yet there is a danger that this may, over time, undermine the broader professional practice community, with its preference for strong forms of discretion, as they become ever more wary of the GMC and its associated bureaucratic machinery (Irvine 2006).

Risk-based regulation, professional discretion and medical game-playing

An apposite example here is the introduction of medical audit in the NHS to support the promotion of good clinical governance and performance management of medical work (McDonald et al 2008). Power emphasises the enormous impact of the contemporary trend in all spheres of Western societies towards audit in all its guises, with its economic concern with transparent accountability and standardisation, particularly for judging the activities of experts (Power 2000). Pertinent data relating to a doctor's professional activities, such as prescribing patterns, the outcomes of case note analysis, the results of clinical audit, as well as patient complaint case outcomes and surgical operation success rates, are all now recorded under the aegis of clinical governance, in order to ensure compliance with best-practice performance frameworks, guidelines and protocols (Bruce 2007).

Yet in his review of the implementation of medical audit, Power discovered that doctors used their esoteric expertise and discretionary professional judgement to resist being 'colonised' by audit, and instead engaged in 'creative compliance and game playing around targets' (Power 2000: 106). Thus, practitioners appeared to incorporate audit into their practice, but in reality continued much the same practices as they had done before. Furthermore, research has found that hospital management were often complicit within this process, as they tended to overlook this game playing by doctors, in case acknowledging it publicly undermined confidence in NHS governance frameworks.

Game playing by doctors in relation to clinical governance performance frameworks, combined with a degree of managerial collusion in such activity, is arguably the dysfunctional consequence of the increasing contemporary reliance on governing tools that emphasise the use of standardised judgements, and therefore weak forms of professional discretion, to ensure greater efficiency, transparency and accountability (Gray and Harrison 2004). Responding by engaging in game playing enables practitioners to appear to have met the formal reporting requirements of transparent quality assurance processes, when they have in fact continued to operate in much the same way they always have done, with the added benefit that their superficial ritualised compliance with this new governing regime has created a more firmly bounded workspace within which to operate without outside interference (Waring 2007a).

Medical revalidation and the risks of risk-based regulation

The response of practitioners to the introduction of medical audit provides an illustrative lesson in how a reliance on risk-averse, codified and routinised frameworks to guide action within healthcare systems can alter the behaviour of the wider professional community in unforeseen ways, as doctors seek to adjust to changing circumstance and to avoid the possibility of punitive action being taken against them (Waring 2007b). In the context of the structure and operational culture of the GMC, there is a danger that the growth of risk-focused forms of medical regulation and regulatory oversight may bring with them unintended negative consequences for patient care and public safety. This is particularly the case given the presence of concerns within the medical profession about reforms to the GMC.

One important area for consideration here is medical revalidation. Revalidation is designed to document how doctors are ensuring that they remain fit to practise in their chosen specialty and involves a thorough assessment of a practitioner, using a mixture of performance appraisals, patient feedback and continuing professional development activities (Donaldson 2008). Only by successfully completing the revalidation process every five years will doctors be able to remain on the medical register and continue to practise medicine. The GMC progressively expanded the coverage of medical revalidation nationally from 2012 onwards (NHS Revalidation Support Team 2014). The next chapter will investigate whether practitioners are responding to the revalidation process in a similar fashion to the way that they have acted towards medical audit and, if so, what the consequences of this might be for the future of both revalidation and the GMC.

Conclusion

Over the last two decades, legislative reform in the regulation of doctors has supported the development of a risk-based model of professional governance, which has prompted fundamental changes in the internal organisational structure of the GMC (Scrivens 2007). The GMC is undoubtedly a very different organisation from what it was previously. No longer is it *the* symbol of medical authority, status and power: the traditional, doctors-only 'club mentality' has shifted to permit the inclusion of non-medical members. Underpinning risk-based regulation is a reliance on formulised 'risk templates', which act as decision-making aids and promote institutional performance appraisal and accountability (Hutter and Power 2005). Consequently, the GMC now possesses open and transparent administrative protocols, processes and outcome measures, from which its operational performance can be measured and judged.

In the past, as a result of high-profile scandals, the GMC has been accused of bias towards doctors and has been criticised for not fulfilling its statutory obligation to protect the public. As a result, it has sought to become more transparent in its operations (Waring and Dixon-Woods 2010). In this context, the notion of institutional transparency can be understood as a policy device designed to enable practices that are open to public scrutiny in order to generate greater trust and legitimacy. Furthermore, the introduction of revalidation and reforms in the hearing of fitness to practise cases are demonstrative of an organisation undergoing a transition from a reactive, incident-led institution that has been preoccupied with ensuring medical privilege, to a proactive overseer of professional standards designed to secure the public interest. It is the focus of subsequent chapters to ascertain whether these developments lend support to the conclusion that the shift towards risk-based regulation better protects the public interest.

References

Allsop, J and Saks, M (2002) *Regulating the Health Professions* (London: Sage)

Bosk, C L (1978) *Forgive and Remember: Managing Medical Failure* (Chicago: University of Chicago Press)

Bristol Royal Infirmary Inquiry (2001) *Learning From Bristol: The Report of the Public Inquiry into Children's Heart Surgery at the Bristol Royal Infirmary, 1984-1995* (London: Stationery Office)

Bruce, D A (2007) Regulation of Doctors, *BMJ*, 334: 436-37

Chamberlain, J M (2012) *The Sociology of Medical Regulation: An Introduction* (NY and Amsterdam: Springer)

Cranberg, L D, Glick, T H and Sato, L (2008) Do the Claims Hold up? A Study of Medical Negligence Claims against Neurologists, *Journal of Empirical Legal Studies*, 4: 155-62.

Department of Health (DOH) (2001) *Harold Shipman's Clinical Practice 1974–1998: A Clinical Audit Commissioned by the Chief Medical Officer* (London: DOH)

Donaldson, L (2008) *Revalidation: Next Steps* (London: DOH)

Dworkin, G (1977) *Taking Rights Seriously* (London: Duckworth)

Evetts, J (2002) New Directions in State and International Professional Occupations: Discretionary Decision-making and Acquired Regulation, *Work, Employment and Society*, 16: 341-53

Freidson, E (2001) *Professionalism: The Third Logic* (Cambridge: Polity Press)

General Medical Council (GMC) (2013) *Raising and Acting on Concerns about Patient* Safety (London: GMC)

Gladstone, D (2000) *Regulating Doctors* (London: Institute for the Study of Civil Society)

Gray, A and Harrison, S (2004) *Governing Medicine: Theory and Practice* (Buckinghamshire: Open University Press)

Hood, C and Miller, P (2010) *Risk and Public Services: Report by the ESRC Centre for Analysis of Risk and Regulation* (London: London School of Economics)

Hutter, B and Power, M (2005) *Organisational Encounters with Risk* (Cambridge: Cambridge University Press)

Irvine, D (2003) *The Doctors' Tale: Professionalism and Public Trust* (Abingdon: Radcliffe Medical Press)

Irvine, D (2006) Success Depends Upon Winning Hearts and Minds, *BMJ*, 333: 965-6.

Jones, I (2011) Still Just Rhetoric? Judicial Discretion and Due Process, *Liverpool Law Review*, 32: 251-73

Kaye, K (2006) Stuck in the Middle: The Rise of the Meso-regulators, *Risk and Regulation*, 6: 23-35

Kuhlmann, E (2006) Traces of Doubt and Sources of Trust: Health Professions in an Uncertain Society, *Current Sociology*, 54: 607-19

Larson, M (1978) *The Rise of Professionalism* (Los Angeles: University of California Press)

Law Commission (2014a) *Regulation of Health Care Professionals, Regulation of Social Care Professionals in England*, Law Commission Consultation Paper No 202 (London: The Law Commission England)

Law Commission (2014b) *Regulation of Health Care Professionals, Regulation of Social Care Professionals in Northern Ireland*, Law Commission Consultation Paper No 12 (Belfast: The Law Commission Northern Ireland)

Law Commission (2014c) *Regulation of Health Care Professionals, Regulation of Social Care Professionals in Scotland*, Scottish Law Commission Discussion Paper No 153 (Edinburgh: The Law Commission Scotland)

Lloyd-Bostock, S (2010) The Creation of Risk-Related Information: The UK General Medical Council's Electronic Database, *Journal of Health Organisation and Management*, 24: 584-96

Lloyd-Bostock, S and Hutter, B M (2008) Reforming Regulation of the Medical Profession: The Risks of Risk-based Approaches, *Health, Risk and Society*, 10: 69-83

Marquand, D (1988) *The Unprincipled Society: New Demands and Old Politics* (London: Jonathon Cape)

McDonald, R, Harrison, S and Checkland, K (2008) Incentives and Control in Primary Health Care: Findings from English Pay-for-Performance Case Studies, *Journal of Health Organisation and Management*, 22: 48-62

Merrison, A (1975) *Committee of Inquiry into the Regulation of the Medical Profession* (London: HMSO)

Moran, M (2004) *Governing Doctors in the British Regulatory State* (Buckinghamshire: Open University Press)

NHS Revalidation Support Team (2014) *The Early Benefits and Impact of Medical Revalidation: Report on Research Findings in Year One* (London: DOH)

Power, M (2000) *The Audit Society: Rituals of Verification* (Oxford: Oxford University Press)

Samanta, A, Mello, M M, Foster, C, Tingle, C and Samanta, J (2006) The Role of Clinical Guidelines in Medical Negligence Litigation: A Shift from the Bolam Standard?, *Medical Law Review*, 14: 321-66

Scrivens, S (2007) The Future of Regulation and Governance, *Journal of the Royal Society for the Promotion of Health*, 127: 72-7

Secretary of State for Health (2007) *Trust, Assurance and Safety – The Regulation of Health Professions in the 21st Century* (London: Stationery Office)

Smith, J (2005) *Shipman: Final Report* (London: DOH)

Smith, R (1998) All Changed, Changed Utterly, *BMJ*, 316:1917-18

Soothill, K and Wilson, D (2005) Theorising the Puzzle that is Harold Shipman, *Journal of Forensic Psychiatry and Psychology*, 16: 685-98

Stacey, M (1992) *Regulating British Medicine* (London: John Wiley and Sons)

Waring, J (2007a) Adaptive Regulation or Governmentality: Patient Safety and the Changing Regulation of Medicine, *Sociology of Health and Illness*, 29: 163-79

Waring, J (2007b) Beyond Blame: The Cultural Barriers to Medical Incident Reporting, *Social Science and Medicine*, 60: 1927-35

Waring, J and Dixon-Woods, M (2010) Modernising Medical Regulation: Where Are We Now?, *Journal of Health Organisation and Management*, 24: 540-55

2

FITNESS TO PRACTISE IN THE WORKPLACE: MEDICAL REVALIDATION

Revalidation will be based on a local evaluation of doctors' practice through appraisal, and its purpose is to affirm good practice. By doing so, it will assure patients and the public, employers, other healthcare providers, and other health professionals that licensed doctors are practising to the appropriate professional standards. It will also complement other systems that exist within organisations and at other levels for monitoring standards of care and recognising and responding to concerns about doctors' practice. (Department of Health (DOH) 2014: 2)

Introduction

Chapter One highlighted that two ideas have long defined the contractual nature of the relationship between the medical profession and the public under the legislative terms of the principle of self-regulation. First is the idea that, as they do an occupation which possesses specialist expertise and a strong ethical 'service orientation', doctors can be left alone to manage their affairs, including the training, monitoring and disciplining of group members. Second is the related idea that, once qualified, a doctor can be left alone to practise until they retire. It also outlined how the shift towards risk-based regulation has led to these two interrelated ideas being challenged, with contemporary reforms to the GMC introducing greater transparency and accountability in the regulation of doctors and how their fitness to practise is ensured. Chapter Two focuses on one of these reforms – medical revalidation. It traces its historical development and implementation as well as critically examining recent research into its application. In doing so, the chapter highlights areas for critical consideration in relation to future policy and practice.

Challenging medicine: the rise of hospital management and the patient revolt

It is often argued that, although it was initially proposed in the 1970s, revalidation began in 2000, when the GMC published a consultation document: *Revalidating Doctors: Ensuring Standards, Securing the Future* (GMC 2000). This document came into being as a result of high-profile medical error and malpractice cases, such as the case of Harold Shipman, who murdered over two hundred of his patients. Yet it is important to note, if only for the sake of holistic clarity, that there was increasing state intervention in the field of medical regulation from the early 1970s onwards, particularly in relation to the operation of the NHS. As well as that, this was in no small part as a result of rapid advances in medical knowledge and technology and a concurrent need, first, to ensure that doctors kept up to date with these developments, and second, to minimise costs and increase service effectiveness.

On creation of the NHS in 1948, the state and the medical profession entered into an agreement that was mutually beneficial – the state obtained a suitability qualified expert workforce and the profession was granted a monopoly over the provision of medical services. The problem was that the concordat between medicine and the state was a product of its time. During the 'consensus politics' era after the

Second World War, the prevailing wisdom was that 'experts know best'. However, by the 1970s, times had changed and the public was gradually becoming less and less willing to accept the authority of experts without question. Furthermore, when the NHS had been founded there was broad cross-party agreement that the welfare state was necessary and that steady economic growth would ensure the progressive decline of poverty and the improvement of public health. But by the late 1960s to early 1970s, growing public expenditure was a very real issue, with both main political parties instigating reviews of public services, particularly in relation to unemployment benefit, social welfare provision and the funding of the NHS.

Certainly, the 1979 Conservative administration, led by Mrs Margaret Thatcher, wished to reduce public expenditure. Thatcherism held a firm ideological commitment to 'rolling back the state' and introducing free market forces in both the public and private spheres. The 1979 Conservative administration's neo-liberal commitment to the discipline of the market and the power of consumer choice meant it perceived all forms of professional self-regulation (and medical autonomy in the NHS in particular) as being opposed to choice and competition. This led to a situation where, although the state was publicly supporting a doctor's right to clinical freedom, it was also calling for NHS reforms to contain costs and improve efficiency. It is against this background that in 1983 the NHS Management Inquiry gave its recommendations (Chamberlain 2012). Roy Griffiths, who was the Managing Director of Sainsbury's supermarket chain, chaired this inquiry. The Griffiths Report, as it subsequently became known, led to the replacement of the traditional medically controlled hospital administrator with general managers (later known as 'chief executives') tasked with ensuring the efficient use of resources. Further NHS reforms initiated by Conservative administrations throughout the 1980s and early 1990s – such as *Working for Patients* (DOH 1989) and *The Patient's Charter* (DOH 1991) – would lead to subsequent challenges to 'doctor power' under the guise of improving efficiency and empowering patients.

By the beginning of the 1990s, NHS management had established control over hospital information systems and clinical budgets, which in themselves meant that managers possessed more control over doctors' clinical activities than any 'outsider' ever had. The state's reforms further expanded management's influence, to include the allocation of merit awards, the appointment of hospital consultants and annual reviews of their job descriptions. Flynn noted that there had been a 'tendency during the last decade … towards an erosion of professional dominance in the face of increased … managerial power' (Flynn 1992: 50).

Increasing public concern with the principle of medical self-regulation was an interwoven theme of NHS reform and the growth of the viewpoint of patient as consumer. Certainly, public suspicion of collegiate control of doctors' discipline came to the foreground in the early 1980s as the GMC's commitment to protecting patients' interests was increasingly questioned in the media. In 1983, Professor Ian Kennedy gave his Reith Lectures called 'The Unmasking of Medicine' (Kennedy 1983). Professor Kennedy criticised the GMC's lack of openness and public accountability. He argued that its disciplinary procedures were not transparent and protected doctors instead of patients. He also called for measures to be introduced that would ensure the continued competence of doctors. Meanwhile, television programmes such as *Dispatches*, *That's Life*, *World in Action* and *File on Four*, repeatedly highlighted cases of medical malpractice and blamed the GMC for failing to ensure that the doctors they investigated were trustworthy and competent (Chamberlain 2012).

The central issue of continuing medical education

By the early 1990s, NHS reforms and the patient revolt had led to the recognition that it simply could no longer be assumed that doctors would remain competent throughout their career without periodically updating their knowledge and skills. There can also be no doubt that the rapidly changing and expanding nature of medical knowledge meant that the elite institutions of the medical profession involved in medical education, such as the Royal Colleges and the GMC, came to recognise by the end of the 1980s that they had to look at this issue, with a view to enhancing both its provision and governance.

This move by the GMC towards looking at doctors' continued competence to practise was progressive. Nevertheless, throughout the 1980s and into the early 1990s it remained an essentially reactive institution, providing little effective leadership to the profession at large. Indeed, it left this up to the British Medical Association (BMA) – the main medical union in the UK – and the Royal Colleges, as it historically had done. It was heavily dependent on building consensus within the profession when deciding policy. It was representing doctors, not regulating them as it should have been, and consequently was perceived by many critical commentators to be failing as a regulatory body in its statutory duty to protect the general public (Gladstone 2000). This situation led the state to feel increasingly justified in developing strategies to monitor (and challenge and change) doctors' clinical activities. For example, by the end of the 1980s, the state was arguing that it was time 'to develop a comprehensive set of measures of the outcome of much of the work of … doctors' (DOH 1989: 2). It had decided 'to consider how the quality of medical care can best be improved by means of medical audit, and on the development of indicators of clinical outcome' (DOH 1989: 2).

First developed in the US to track quality through analysing treatment outcomes, and endorsed by the BMA as a strategy to protect professional autonomy, medical audit seemed to be the perfect tool the state needed to place doctors under greater surveillance and control. The problem was, as a study published at the time indicated, 'rank and file' doctors may 'regard overall financial limitations as being legitimate restrictions on their autonomy … [but do] … not see a legitimate role for peer review or quality assurance' (Harrison and Schultz 1989: 203). The Royal Colleges were ever aware of the turning political tide and had joined the BMA in viewing medical audit and peer review as a legitimate way of improving doctor performance, while at the same time retaining medical autonomy. By the early 1990s, they were actively involved in promoting medical audit to the 'rank and file' of the profession (Hopkins 1990). The state needed such allies to make its reforms work and consequently had to accede to the view of medical audit possessed by the Royals Colleges and BMA. Namely, if medical audit was going to be used more frequently and formally, then it should follow what Pollitt (1993) called 'the medical model'. This meant that its operation remained firmly in the hands of doctors themselves, who would periodically advise management on outcomes as they saw fit.

However, this was not the end of the matter. By the end of the 1980s, technological developments like the computer had become more firmly linked to existing statistical and epidemiological techniques. This had led to a rapid increase in the ability to manage and analyse clinical outcomes and to establish 'low risk' guidelines and protocols for doctors to follow (Wennberg 1988). As the 1990s progressed, the state would move towards introducing multidisciplinary clinical audit and proactively sought to develop risk management strategies across professional groups (NHS Executive 1994). While the use of medical audit and clinical audit was on the rise, evidence-based medicine was also developing to address regional variations in key performance outcome areas, such as mortality rates following surgery and length of stay in hospital following admission (Berg 1997). Some were worried that this would lead to the establishment of 'cook book medicine'. Evidence-based medicine not only promised to help the state to place medical work under greater surveillance, but it also promised to help patients make more informed choices with regard to treatment.

Finally, a mixture of political will and modern technology was supporting changes in the nature of the doctor–patient power relationship. As Wennberg noted at the time:

> [It] is now possible to speak of a new set of disciplines which together constitute the evaluative clinical sciences. They offer the promise of a scientific programme that can greatly improve clinical decision-making by decreasing uncertainty about the probabilities and the value to patients of the outcomes of care. They also offer new ways of communicating information to physicians and patients that can greatly increase understanding

about the consequences of medical choices and thus help patients make decisions they truly want. (Wennberg 1988: 34)

Introducing doctor appraisal

To summarise, by the mid-to-late 1990s, peer and managerial surveillance of individual doctor's clinical activities had become the norm under the banner of promoting cost-efficiency, reducing risk and ensuring patient involvement in medical decision-making. The rapid development in clinical guidelines and protocols to govern the performance of doctors and other healthcare staff was seen by many interested observers to be a consequence of the rise of the idea of patient as consumer. For example, Allsop and Mulcahy (1996) held the increasingly common view among commentators that there was an expanding web of formal rules (guidelines and protocols) as well as informal rules (norms of behaviour held by an individual healthcare actor's social networks) – operating both internally and externally to the medical profession itself – which were increasingly governing the day-to-day activities of individual doctors. This state of affairs, they felt, was a result of new relationships being forged between what they held to be the four main stakeholders involved in healthcare – government, citizens, managers and professionals.

The introduction of annual appraisal was held by many to be symbolic of this new state of affairs. The publication of *The NHS Plan* in 2000 highlighted that the purpose of annual appraisal was to support doctors to maintain 'medical excellence' (DOH 2000). The BMA negotiated with the state an agreement whereby annual appraisal (which was finally introduced nationally in 2003) would be a formative developmental educational exercise, undertaken with another doctor, and ordered in line with the principles of good clinical governance and the GMC's *Good Medical Practice* (GMC 2013a). In other words, although in principle and in practice open to managerial input and review, annual appraisal would essentially be doctor controlled. Furthermore, it would not lead to extreme punitive action against the doctor in question, such as removal from the medical register. Every year a doctor would maintain a portfolio of evidence of their activities and achievements. This would contain, for example, an overview of teaching and clinical duties, prescribing lists, clinical guidelines used and results of trust clinical governance reviews (including, for instance, a doctor's surgical success:failure ratio), certificates of attendance to Royal College continuing professional development (CPD) courses and specialty conferences, feedback from colleagues, as well as patient feedback or complaints. A Royal College trained colleague would review this portfolio evidence, to identify developmental needs for the next year.

Medicine's new professionalism and the beginnings of medical revalidation

Annual appraisal was built on the recognition that throughout the 1990s, the Royal Colleges had gradually introduced more and more formal arrangements for ensuring a doctor's CPD (Chamberlain 2012). They worked with the BMA, NHS management and the state to establish mechanisms whereby sanctions were introduced for doctors who failed to gain CPD 'points' for completing college courses, such as exclusion from merit awards and the supervision of junior doctor training posts. However, these lacked the key sanction possessed solely by the GMC: removal from the medical register for non-completion of CPD. In summary, while medicine's elites recognised that something needed to be done to ensure that doctors remained up to date and fit to practise in their chosen specialty, a tendency towards mutual protectionism could be said to still be in operation.

Not all the critical voices belonged to individuals outside the profession. There had always been reformer voices within the profession demanding that the GMC become more proactive and take up the challenge of underperforming doctors and ensuring that practitioners remained fit to practise. Particularly among general practitioners, but also from powerful 'in house' commentators such as Richard Smith, who was editor of the prestigious publication the *British Medical Journal* (Smith 1992). Medical reformers felt that the

GMC was too far removed from the needs of the profession. They wanted it to provide definitive leadership to its 'rank and file' members, by forging a more open and accountable relationship with the public. One of these reformers, who was heavily influenced by the sociologist and GMC lay member Margaret Stacey as well as the eminent medical sociologist Margot Jeffreys, was a general practitioner called Dr Donald Irvine (now Sir Donald Irvine). When elected in 1995, he would be the first leader of the GMC to be a general practitioner since its foundation 137 years previously. Irvine noted:

> In 1995, I stood for election as President of the GMC, on a programme of reform both of professionalism in medicine and the GMC itself. There were members within the GMC, both medical and lay, who believed that such reform of the GMC had to be carried out swiftly. Otherwise public confidence in the medical profession, and in particular in the system of professional self-regulation, for which the GMC was primarily responsible, could not be sustained. (Irvine 2003: 11)

The foundation stone of Irvine's new professionalism was the recognition that self-regulation was a privilege not an inherent right. Hence, the number of lay members of the GMC was increased. He also advocated the establishment of clear standards that could be operationalised into outcomes for assessment. Between 1992 and 1995, the GMC sought and took highly progressive steps to assume legislative powers to assess doctors' performance through the Medical (Professional Performance) Act 1995. This led to the publication in 1995 of the first edition of *Good Medical Practice* (GMC 2013a), which listed the principal attributes of good medical practice under seven headings:

1. Good clinical care;
2. Maintaining good medical practice;
3. Relationships with patients;
4. Teaching and training, appraising and assessing;

5. Working with colleagues;
6. Probity;
7. Health.

Good Medical Practice has been subject to change over the years and the current version (GMC 2013a) divides these attributes into four competency domains:

- Domain 1: Knowledge, skills and performance;
- Domain 2: Safety and quality;
- Domain 3: Communication, partnership and teamwork;
- Domain 4: Maintaining trust.

A further publication, *Duties of a Doctor* (GMC 1995), placed respect for patients and the need to maintain clinical competence at the centre of medical professionalism. The publication of these two documents was the first sign that the growing culture of standard setting and performance appraisal in the NHS was reaching medicine's own professional institutions. A key part of Irvine's reforms included the revision of the GMC's new performance procedures, which involved developing appraisal instruments. These operationalised *Good Medical Practice* into key competency domains, whereby assessors could mark a doctor's 'on-the-job' performance. The scheme's appraisal instruments were subsequently published in the academic journal *Medical Education* (Southgate 2001). The scheme was linked to the final part of Irvine's reform agenda, which was to push for the introduction of the periodic recertification of a doctor's 'fitness to practise' to stay on the medical register (known as 'medical revalidation'). But then the events of the respective Shipman and Bristol Royal Infirmary cases (outlined in Chapter One) happened, and in the words of Richard Smith (1998), it became a situation where everything 'changed, changed utterly'.

Bristol and Shipman: all changed, changed utterly

Bristol made the GMC realise its plans for medical revalidation needed to go ahead at pace. The consultation process started in 1998 with various stakeholders, such as the BMA and patient support groups, attending a GMC conference on the topic (Chamberlain 2012). The process was heated with debate raging over whether revalidation was needed, and if so, what form it should take. Members of the public wanted revalidation and voiced the need for it. Conversely, there were 'rank and file' members of the profession and members of its elite institutions, which under no circumstances wanted a periodic exam to form the basis for revalidation. The BMA's Hospital Consultants and Specialists Committee (HCSC) argued against revalidation because of the time and expense it would involve. The Royal Colleges and GMC were for it. In 1999 it was decided that 'to maintain their registration, all doctors must be able to demonstrate regularly that they continue to be fit to practise in their chosen specialty' (GMC 1999: 1).

What had to be decided would be the form that revalidation would take. A further period of consultation was entered into to decide this. The GMC wanted regional centers to undertake revalidation locally. However, this idea was dismissed by the BMA as impractical. The GMC knew it had to move quickly. As part of its reforms of the NHS and because of the problems highlighted by Bristol the Department of Health had published *Supporting Doctors, Protecting Patients* (DOH 1999). This proposed that all doctors undergo an Annual Appraisal as part of their NHS contract. As already noted, the publication the next year of the *NHS Plan* formally introduced appraisal (DOH 2000).

Although not originally intended to link with revalidation it was generally agreed by 2001 that the successful completion of five Annual Appraisals, after external review by two medical and one lay GMC assessors, would in itself be enough for the purposes of revalidation (Gentleman 2001). Though it clearly had merits, this proposed method of revalidation was 'lightweight' compared to the original intention of establishing regional revalidation 'centres' to undertake pass/fail tests of doctor's competence. Yet it never got off the ground due to the case of serial killer, Harold Shipman, a general practitioner in Hyde, Greater Manchester.

Dr Shipman was a popular doctor, well respected by his patients. Between 1995 and 1998, he murdered 15 elderly patients with lethal doses of diamorphine. Subsequently, it was discovered that between 1974 and 1998 he had murdered 215 patients (all elderly) and doubts remained about a further 45 (Smith 2005). The police informed the GMC they were investigating Dr Shipman in 1998 and he was subsequently convicted of murder in 2000. It was only after his conviction that he was stuck off the medical register.

Similar to the Bristol case, the Shipman case caused a public outcry. It was discovered that Shipman had previously been before the GMC's disciplinary committee in 1976 for dishonestly obtaining drugs and forging NHS prescriptions. He had been dealt with leniently and essentially 'let off' with a warning.

This signaled the start of another period of intense criticism for the GMC. The state ordered a public inquiry into the Shipman case, chaired by Dame Janet Smith. As the Secretary of State, Mr Milburn, made it clear at the time: 'The GMC … must be truly accountable and it must be guided at all times by the welfare and safety of patients. We owe it to the relatives of Shipman's victims to prevent a repetition of what happened in Hyde' (quoted in Gladstone 2000: 10).

During the Shipman Inquiry, the GMC made changes to its membership. A new GMC was launched in 2003, just after Irvine's reign as president ended. The GMC's executive membership was reduced, 40% of whom were lay members. In February 2003, Professor Sir Graeme Catto took over from Irvine as president of the GMC. Like Irvine before him, Catto continued to maintain its professionally led medical regulation, based on an open and accountable partnership with patients, which best protects the public interest (Catto 2006 2007). The GMC continued with its plans for revalidation during this time. Indeed Catto wrote to doctors in 2003 telling them to 'get ready' for revalidation (Chamberlain 2012). However, the GMC's revalidation plans were to all intents and purposes deliberately slowed down until Dame Janet Smith published her full report in January 2005.

In her report, Smith (2005) highlighted key lessons that needed to be taken on board by the NHS and the medical profession in relation to topics such as the checking of death certificates, scrutiny of single-handed GP practices and the monitoring of death rates and medical records. About the proposal that five Annual Appraisals would equal revalidation, Smith (2005: 1048) felt that this would not have identified Shipman and did 'not offer the public protection from underperforming doctors'. She highlighted that the formative nature of Annual Appraisal meant that it was unsuitable for use as a summative pass/fail examination tool, as required by Revalidation. She felt that instead of taking a strong stance, as required of it as a regulatory body, the GMC had essentially caved in to pressure from within the profession to abandon its original idea of independent regional revalidation 'centres'.

That is, the possibility of 'summative pass/fail testing had been dropped in favour of a 'light-touch' approach to revalidation that essentially involved 'rubber stamping' existing Annual Appraisals. Indeed, Smith (2005: 1174) said that the GMC's original 'proposals were unpopular with a powerful section of the profession. So the GMC retreated from its earlier vision and devised a system that it calls revalidation but which does not involve any evaluation of a doctor's fitness to practise'. Concerned about the GMC's move away from adopting a more rigorous approach to revalidation, she actively criticised Catto's comparison of it to an MOT on a BBC radio programme. She said:

> He [Sir Catto] expressed pride in the fact that no other country in the world had a system of time-limited licence dependent upon doctors demonstrating they are up to date and fit to practise. To call revalidation an MOT for doctors is a catchword. It is easy for the listener to remember. I think that many people who heard that programme would have taken away the impression that revalidation is a test for doctors, just like the MOT. That is not a true impression. (Smith 2005: 1086)

A culture of medical protectionism?

About the working culture of the GMC, Smith (2005) echoed the voices of many observers in feeling that although the GMC had changed it had not changed enough:

> I would like to believe that the GMCs working culture would continue to change in the right direction by virtue of its own momentum. However, I do not feel confident it will do so. I am sure they are many people within the GMC, both members and staff, who want to see the regulation of the medical profession based upon the principles of 'patient centred' medicine and public protection. The problem seems to be that, when specific issues arise, opposing views are taken, and as in the past, the balance sometimes tips in the interests of doctors. (Smith 2005: 1176)

Furthermore, Smith (2005) discussed how the elected nature of medical members on the GMC made the central issue of protecting the interests of the public difficult for members:

> it seems ... that one of the fundamental problems facing the GMC is the perception, shared by many doctors, that it is supposed to be 'representing' them. It is not, it is regulating them. ... In fact the medical profession has a very effective representative body in the BMA, it does not need – and should not have – two. (Smith 2005: 1176)

Her recommendation was that the makeup of the GMC be changed so elected members were replaced with nominated members, selected by the Privy Council via the Public Appointees Committee after a period of 'open competition' on the basis of their ability to serve the public interest. Smith (2005: 1174) concluded that she was 'driven to the conclusion that, for the majority of GMC members, the old culture of protecting the interests of doctors lingers on'.

The Health and Social Care Act 2008 and medical revalidation

What became clear after the publication of the Shipman Report was that the criticisms regarding the GMC's working culture and proposals for revalidation meant the state had to step in and undertake a full review of medical regulation. The then Health Secretary, John Reid, commissioned the then Chief Medical Officer, Sir Liam Donaldson, to undertake the review. His subsequent report was published in July 2006 (Donaldson 2006) and informed the content of the Health and Social Care Act 2008. The Act introduced several key reforms in medical regulation. Non-medical lay members now have to make up half of the GMC membership. Furthermore an independent system overseen by the Public Appointments Commission was introduced to elect GMC members, while the grounds on which fitness to practise panels (FPPs) operate was also changed. As already noted in Chapter One, such cases whereby a practitioner's fitness to practise is called into question have traditionally been judged on the criminal standard: beyond all reasonable doubt – a situation that frequently led commentators to argue that the GMC's disciplinary procedures first and foremost protected doctors. But the 2008 Act required that such cases now be judged on the civil standard of proof: on the balance of probability. It was argued that this will enable underperforming doctors to be more easily stopped from practising medicine. To enhance impartiality and the independence of the case hearing process, the 2008 Act also required cases to be heard by an independent adjudicator, not by members of the GMC. This latter point was particularly contentious and what actually happened next will be discussed at length in Chapter Three, which explores FPP reforms in detail.

Chapter One noted how the 2008 Act is symbolic of the emergence of a risk-based approach to professional regulation in the UK, at the centre of which lies the recognition of the need to utilise risk templates and multiple data-points to identify, manage and minimise risk threats (Lloyd-Bostock and Hutter 2008). In the context of medical revalidation, the 2008 Act was built on the recognition of the need to use best-evidenced clinical governance frameworks and outcomes to measure and judge medical performance, as well as of the need for greater managerial, patient and interprofessional involvement in revalidation. After a period of consultation with government, the NHS, the BMA, the Royal Colleges, and the general public, revalidation was implemented nationally by the GMC in a staged format between 2012 and 2016. In its post-Donaldson finalised guise, revalidation is essentially made up of two elements – relicensing and recertification – which incorporate NHS appraisal within them.

Relicensing seeks to make current NHS appraisal arrangements more rigorous, with greater direct testing of a doctor's competence with regard to key day-to-day clinical tasks. To stay on the medical register, all doctors will now have to successfully pass the relicensing requirement that they have successfully completed five NHS annual performance appraisals. Specialist recertification will also occur every five years. It will involve a thorough 'hands on' assessment of a doctor, organised and quality assured by a doctor's peers and associated professional associations. Although the resulting finalised process and language used to describe it differ somewhat from Donaldson's, it is nevertheless the case that the 2008 Act signified *on paper* that there has been a shift towards a more robust and rigorous system than was envisaged by medical elites at the beginning of the new millennium.

Responsible officers: implementing revalidation at a local level

The Health and Social Care Act 2008 introduced what was called a 'GMC affiliate', who was later known as a 'responsible officer' (RO). This person operates at a local NHS level, to coordinate the revalidation of practitioners. The exact arrangements for this process were defined by the Medical Profession (Responsible Officers) Regulations 2010 and 2013, which also set out the requirements for professional oversight of the process. From April 2013 a new body, NHS England, was given responsibility for the RO role that previously was the responsibility of strategic health authorities and primary care trusts. As a result, ROs for doctors in England now have a prescribed connection to NHS England, while the remaining ROs are connected to either

Health Education England, NHS Education for Scotland, the Health Departments in England and Scotland or the Welsh Government (DOH 2014).

ROs work within what are referred to as 'designated bodies' (that is, employing organisations), which have overall responsibility for revalidation. An RO must, at the time of appointment, must have been fully registered with the GMC for the previous five years. Hence, given its recent implementation, they must have held a licence to practise from the time when medical revalidation was formally introduced in 2012. They must also complete a GMC and Royal College approved introductory training programme for ROs within 12 months of appointment. Medical practitioners in the UK only have one designated body and one RO, irrespective of how many organisations they are contractually employed to. The specific responsibilities of an RO are (BMA 2015):

- ensuring that effective systems to support revalidation are in place (including appraisal and clinical governance systems);
- evaluating the fitness to practise of all doctors with whom the designated body has a prescribed connection and making a recommendation to the GMC regarding revalidation;
- identifying and investigating concerns about doctors' conduct or performance;
- ensuring that support and remediation are provided where a doctor's practice falls below the required standard;
- overseeing doctors whose practice is supervised or limited under conditions imposed by the GMC.

ROs make recommendations to the GMC about a doctor's fitness to practise. Their recommendation will be based on the outcome of annual appraisals over a five-year period, combined with information drawn from the organisational clinical governance systems (for example, surgical operation rates). To this end, practitioners are required to maintain a personal portfolio of their fitness to practise, which contains in it evidence that they have met the competency domain requirements set out in *The Good Medical Practice Framework for Appraisal and Revalidation* (GMC 2014; see Appendix One). This lists required evidence within the four domains of *Good Medical Practice* (GMC 2013a):

1. Knowledge, skills and performance;
2. Safety and quality;
3. Communication, partnership and teamwork;
4. Maintaining trust.

In its 'end-user' document *Revalidation: What You Need to Do* (GMC 2013b), the GMC outlines how each practitioner must demonstrate that they have collected and reflected on the following:

- continuing professional development;
- quality improvement activity;
- significant events;
- feedback from colleagues;
- feedback from patients;
- review of complaints and compliments.

Based on the evidence presented, ROs can make one of the following three recommendations to the GMC concerning a doctor's revalidation (BMA 2015):

- **A positive recommendation:** this means that the RO believes that the doctor is up to date, fit to practise and should be revalidated In order to have a positive recommendation, it is mandatory that the doctor has engaged with revalidation processes.
- **Request a deferral:** this could be because the RO needs more information to make a recommendation about the doctor. This might happen if the doctor has taken a break from their practice (for example, maternity or sick leave).
- **Non-engagement:** this is when the RO believes that a doctor has failed to participate in the local systems or processes (such

as appraisal) that support revalidation. The GMC defines non-engagement as: 'A doctor is not engaging in revalidation where, in the absence of reasonable circumstances, they: i) do not participate in the local processes and systems that support revalidation on an ongoing basis and or ii) do not participate in the formal revalidation process.' This recommendation is taken very seriously and can result in the removal of the licence to practise. Engagement in the process by the individual is absolutely crucial in order to avoid this recommendation.

Based on the recommendation it receives from the RO, the GMC will then make the final decision on whether the doctor can retain their licence to practise. It is undoubtedly the case that *on paper*, revalidation involves a thorough assessment of a doctor's fitness to practise using a mixture of appraisals, patient feedback and CPD activities. It is not too difficult to conclude, therefore, that revalidation transforms the GMC from an incident-led, reactive regulatory institution to a proactive overseer of a rolling programme of performance review.

Non-medical input is essential to the revalidation process. Peer-based standard setting and performance assessment – via medical colleagues (in this case, the RO) and professional associations and regulatory bodies using established occupational indicators of good professional practice (in this case, the GMC) – is still acknowledged, by both medical and non-medical observers alike, as *the* essential mechanism by which an individual doctor's clinical competence can be legitimately assessed and underperformance addressed (Irvine 2003).

As a result, revalidation can be said to have come about because contemporary challenges to professional autonomy have brought to the foreground the fact that the principle of medical self-regulation was first institutionalised in the form of the GMC by the Medical Act 1858, as it provided a workable solution to the complex problem of 'how to [both] nurture and control occupations with complex, esoteric knowledge and skill ... which provide us with critical personal services' (Freidson 2001: 220). The changes to the GMC and medical regulation over the last four decades, traced in this and the previous chapter, reinforce that there has been a move towards risk-based regulatory frameworks to better protect the public interest, while at the same time seeking a better balance between 'nurture' and 'control' (Chamberlain 2012).

However, revalidation is undoubtedly a highly contested product and process, the outcomes of which possess implications for the principle of medical autonomy and practitioners and their professional association's traditional control over judgements pertaining to the quality of their practices. This may explain why practitioners and their professional associations resisted its implementation for so long. Initial pilot research into its implementation has revealed that doctors frequently subvert its aims and objectives, processes and outcomes, often claiming as they do so that revalidation seeks to codify and routinise medical decision-making and practitioner clinical performance, when the real world of medical practice is inherently situational, contingent and messy. The rest of this chapter examines this point, in order to more fully establish the impact of the implementation of revalidation on the 'rank and file' members of the medical profession.

Medical revalidation: a Foucauldian interpretation

The fact that revalidation is being introduced in a staged process between 2012 and 2016 means that currently there is minimal information regarding its practical impact on the day-to-day practices of doctors. What does exist will undoubtedly suffer from being somewhat episodic, as not all doctors will have undergone the process – and even those who have done so will only have completed a maximum of one revalidation round. Arguably it will be over a decade before its operation and impact can be fully evaluated. However, some initial investigatory research has been conducted and additionally there is pertinent relevant research relating to the implementation of portfolio-based forms of performance appraisal within the medical profession – annual appraisal.

Paper-based and electronic portfolios are now used throughout medical school and junior doctor training, in later specialist training, as well as to support the implementation of annual appraisal and revalidation of doctors as part of their NHS contract (Snadden and Thomas 1998, Wilkinson et al 2002, Chamberlain 2012). Many things are called portfolios, including logbooks of activity, observational check lists, records of critical incidents and collections of personal reflective narratives (Redman 1995). In line with vocational and professional education in general, a portfolio is typically defined within medicine as a 'dossier of evidence collected over time that demonstrate[s] a doctor's education and practice achievements' (Wilkinson et al 2002: 371). In the context of revalidation, the GMC (2012) currently lists six types of supporting information, which should be present within a doctor's portfolio:

1. continuing professional development (CPD);
2. quality improvement activity;
3. significant events analysis;
4. feedback from colleagues;
5. feedback from patients;
6. complaints and compliments.

The introduction of portfolio-based performance appraisal within medicine presents a significant development in the governance of doctors and the regulation of medical expertise. Indeed, in Chapter One it was argued that it was synergistic with the development of a risk-based approach to professional regulation and forms of neoliberal governance more generally (Lloyd-Bostock and Hutter 2008). It certainly can be argued that the introduction of portfolio-based performance appraisal for doctors is just one more example of the internationally recognised trend that, like many other professionals, doctors are becoming subject to – a seemingly ever increasing number of formal calculative regimes, which seek to performance manage their work practices in order to better economise and risk manage occupational tasks (Coburn and Willis 2000, Checkland et al 2007, McDonald et al 2008).

Power (2007) emphasises the enormous impact of the contemporary trend in all spheres of Western societies towards audit in all its guises – with its economic concern with transparent accountability and standardisation – particularly for judging the activities of experts in order to better minimise risk. This is bound up with the re-emergence of liberalism as an economic and political philosophy (Rose 2000). Against this background, Townley (1993a, 1993b), Newton and Findley (1996) and Chamberlain (2009) all suggest that performance appraisal (portfolio-based or otherwise) is a distinctive form of neoliberal governmentality. That is, it is a system of control which utilises surveillance and rationality to turn the object of its gaze into a calculable and administrable subject that is open to control and risk management (Foucault 1991).

This Foucauldian interpretation of appraisal holds that it acts as an 'information panopticon', which operates through the use of two key panoptic disciplinary mechanisms: normalisation and hierarchy (Zuboff 1988). Normalisation, or normalising judgements, involves comparing, differentiating and homogenising in relation to assumed norms or standards of what is proper, reasonable, desirable and efficient. Appraisal possesses normalising judgements due to its focus on establishing behavioural norms in the form of 'on the job' task standards from which to judge individual performance. Hierarchy involves a process of judging, ranking and rating an individual without in turn being judged. This reinforces that no matter how much its advocates hold that it is user-centred and developmental, performance appraisal is nevertheless a punitive disciplinary tool, concerned with identifying areas of underperformance and correcting them (Fletcher 1997).

Yet appraisal is not a straightforward punitive disciplinary tool, concerned with identifying and correcting poor performance 'from the outside'. Indeed, the Foucauldian interpretation of appraisal holds that it may seek to promote and reward certain behaviours and rectify others, but it recognises that it nevertheless – more often than not – does so by operating using a more subtle and invasive form of soft power (Rose 2000). Certainly, within medicine appraisal seeks to work on the subjectivity of appraisees 'at a distance', through requiring that they engage in self-surveillance of their clinical performance as if it were a normal and everyday practice as a result of the availability of best-evidenced clinical guidelines and protocols (Sheaff et al 2003). For example, for annual NHS appraisal, consultants and general practitioners must keep a portfolio of their CPD needs and fitness to practise, which contains personalised information relating to prescribing patterns, the outcomes of case note analysis, the results of clinical audit, as well as patient complaint case outcomes and surgical operation success rates. They must use this information to help identify and publicly record areas of developmental need in relation to best-practice performance frameworks, guidelines and protocols.

Furthermore, they must subsequently record activities and achievements that demonstrate they are proactively meeting their 'self-identified' learning goals, which will subsequently be subject to formal peer review, to prove that they are willing as a matter of good professionalism to admit to areas of poor performance and to learn from them (Irvine 2003). It will perhaps come as no great surprise, then, to learn that individuals who advocate portfolio-based performance appraisal within medicine argue that it simply formalises what should already be a normal and natural part of a doctor's day-to-day self-monitoring of their clinical performance (see, for example, Snadden and Thomas 1998, Wilkinson et al 2002).

Appraising performance appraisal in medicine

It is certainly the case that research into the growing use of portfolio-based appraisal within medicine provides an invaluable opportunity to examine the positive impact of contemporary reforms in the performance management of medical work. For example, research by West et al (2002), Overeem (2007) Finlay and McLaren (2009) and Brennan et al (2014), among others, reinforces that although it is not possible to objectively establish a direct causal link between appraisal processes and outcomes with improvements (or otherwise) in patient care, there is nevertheless evidence to suggest that medical practitioners have been known to self-report satisfaction with appraisal processes, as well as to claim that it helps them to make positive improvements in their professional practice and their self-management of the continuing fitness to practise.

However, contrasting research does exist. With Redman et al (2000), Smith (2005), Checkland et al (2007) and Chamberlain (2009) have all noted that appraisal processes possess a tendency to operate superficially within medicine. They argue that doctors tend to engage in creative game playing towards appraisals procedural requirements and performance targets, and furthermore, when questioned on this, they tend to rhetorically deploy their specialist esoteric expertise to both normalise and justify their actions (Freidson 2001). Townley (1999) acknowledges that professionals tend to use the personal tacit foundations of their expertise, which is grounded in experiential learning from day-to-day practical professional experience of dealing with patients 'on the shop floor', to 'trump' the rationality of appraisal's information panopticon, as it seeks to construct them as a knowable, calculable and administrable subject.

A key consequence of this is that professional practitioners are able to appear to have met the formal reporting requirements of transparent performance management and quality assurance processes, but have in fact continued to operate in much the same way they always have done. The added benefit is that their superficial, ritualised compliance with this new governing regime has created a more firmly bounded work space within which to operate without outside interference. For example, Chamberlain (2009) found that the practitioners he interviewed fell into one of three camps – 'non-compliers', 'minimalists' and 'enthusiasts':

• Non-compliers did not engage with the process. These individuals may be passionate about their medical specialty and the supervision of trainees, but they nevertheless said that they ignored the portfolio appraisal process evidence when assessing them. Instead, they used traditional teaching and assessment methods (for example ward rounds) and devised their own personalised tests, to assure themselves of a practitioner's competence. The portfolio paperwork was by and large 'fudged' afterwards.

- Similarly, minimalists would fudge the paperwork, but to lesser a degree, as they did utilise some elements of the portfolio appraisal process and evidence, when it came to assessing competence.
- Finally, the enthusiasts, as might be expected, are fully engaged with the appraisal process. However, most importantly, although they rhetorically enthused about the process and used portfolio documents to inform and guide them, like non-compliers and minimalists, enthusiasts reserved the right to exercise their discretion to assess others (in this case, medical students, junior doctors and more senior house officers) as and how they thought fit.

As a result of these findings, Chamberlain (2009) developed the concept of *paperwork compliance* to encapsulate the operation of portfolio-based performance appraisal within medicine. Paperwork compliance exists when the paperwork completion requirements of appraisal are fulfilled, with relevant sections of a portfolio completed and an appraisee 'signed off' by their appraiser as either having met minimum performance criteria or not. However, though the paperwork has been completed, the technical aspects of the appraisal procedures have not been adhered to by the appraiser; that is beyond a highly superficial tick-box, paper-filling level. Chamberlain (2010) notes that:

> Stated in formal terms, *paperwork compliance* gives the impression that an appraisee has been appraised using collegially agreed minimum performance standards. These have been predefined with regards to occupational specific knowledge, skills and attitudinal competency domains. Yet, in reality these have played a superficial role in helping an appraiser form an opinion in regards to: a) Which tasks an appraisee should undertake and be assessed in to be defined as 'competent' at a level appropriate to their career level (that is, compare a final year medical student and a senior house officer); and b) The level of proficiency possessed by an appraisee about these tasks. (Chamberlain 2010: 111)

Chamberlain goes on to illustrate the concept of paperwork compliance using an account from one of his interviewees:

> The following comments from Dr Lime (Physician) encapsulate 'paperwork compliance' succinctly: "Its like this, you fill in the forms in a workmanlike 'dot[t]ing the I's and crossing the T's', fashion. But its all for the look of the thing. It doesn't mean that you actually have done what you are meant to have done, or for that matter believe in what you have written past a very superficial level. You see, you tend to 'bend' the paperwork because you have checked out that everything is OK your own way. So you are just complying with the bureaucratic need to get the paperwork done, and that's all really'. (Chamberlain 2010: 111)

Revalidation: a ritual of employment?

A Foucauldian interpretation of appraisal holds that it acts as an information panopticon, constantly surveying, gathering up and processing appraisees as it seeks to make them ever more calculable and efficient. However, the concept of paperwork compliance draws attention to the fact, well recognised in the performance appraisal literature, that 'if appraisals fail to meet their manifest purpose, they succeed rather as rituals of employment' (Pym 1973: 233). In the sense that appraisal may appear to been carried out occurred on paper, but in reality it has been nothing but an elaborate tick-box exercise. Consequently, it seems to have failed to achieve its manifest panoptic purpose of ensuring worker productivity, organisational efficiency and institutional transparency and accountability.

Research conducted into their perceptions and experience of revalidation has certainly highlighted that many practitioners hold similar views of it as they do of portfolio-based forms of appraisal within medicine more generally. For example, research commissioned by the DOH's own Revalidation Support Team identified a hierarchy in engagement with appraisal and revalidation, with least support from 'rank and file' doctors, more support from trained appraisers and most support from ROs (NHS Revalidation Support Team 2014). A similar disconnection was seen in the perceived value of patient involvement in appraisal.

As revalidation focuses on doctors meeting minimal standards of practice and ongoing education, there is a real need to establish its impact on the culture and behaviours of doctors, including their willingness to identify and seek action on adverse aspects of their own and colleagues' performance and conduct. In this regard, research has highlighted that 65% of appraisers said that they had been able to identify and agree specific circumstances in which doctors they appraised could deliver better care or treatment to patients, but that only 24% of doctors reported that they had changed aspects of their clinical practice or behaviour as a result of their last appraisal (Brennan et al 2014).

Additionally, independent research by the National Centre for Social Research (2014: 2) found that the majority of doctors thought revalidation would be of some value to the profession (59%); however, fewer doctors overall thought revalidation was of value to them personally (51%), or was of value for patient safety (51%). Similarly, independent research by the King's Fund (2014: 1) found that: 'doctors were receiving mixed messages about the purpose of revalidation. All could identify potential benefits, particularly the developmental opportunities. However, there was some cynicism about the overarching purpose of assuring the public of doctors' fitness to practise.'

It is important to note that instances of end-user cynicism, disengagement and manipulation of portfolio-based performance appraisal processes within medicine – be it in relation to junior doctor appraisal, house officer appraisal, annual appraisal for consultants and GPs, or medical revalidation – could be red herrings when it comes to examining their impact on professional practice and organisational working culture. This is not least because these responses are likely to occur in any governmental system of professional performance surveillance and quality assurance (Rose 2000). Certainly, the 'frontstage' and 'backstage' activity and game-playing associated with the concept of paperwork compliance is to be expected, given the esoteric practice-based nature of modern medical expertise and the resulting occupational culture, which reinforces the practical value of nurturing professional autonomy and discretion (Freidson 2001). Furthermore, it certainly is the case that, given time, procedural and outcome mechanisms can be put into place to capture and address end-user cynicism, disengagement and manipulation, with a view to enhancing quality assurance processes and mechanisms (Smither and London 2009). Could the focus on the initial individual response to revalidation to evaluate the success or otherwise of its implementation perhaps therefore be more than a little problematic, particularly given that we are still in the early stages of its operation?

Conclusion: appraising the system

Foucault (1991) himself argued convincingly that the performance appraisal systems and processes bound up with the emergence of modern neoliberal forms of governmentality can never fully capture the inherent contingency and messiness of individual human behaviour and everyday social interaction within complex social systems. It is not the accuracy of the systems in capturing the object of their surveillance, but rather their legitimacy as governing tools in the eyes of social and political elites *and* the masses, which Foucault noted enabled them to continue to operate as mechanisms for social organisation and control. After all, no form of regulation and governance is perfect, and furthermore, it is often regarded as being the fault of the individual and their attitudes and behaviour, rather than the imperfect system, when things go awry – particularly in Western societies, with their inherent focus on individual choice and liberty (Rose 2000).

Given this, what is arguably most important, at least in terms of the issue of ensuring that revalidation enhances the protection of the public from underperforming doctors, is not the presence of end-user cynicism, disengagement or manipulation in relation to revalidation and its current gradual implementation nationwide in the UK; rather, it is the fact that currently there is little objective evidence that practitioner-based performance appraisal *systems* within healthcare – of which revalidation is an example – directly result in improvements in the quality of patient treatment and care (Mugweni et al 2011, Brennan 2014). Therefore, although a research and evaluation focus on individual and localised groups of practitioners is somewhat to be expected (and necessary), arguably the main critical-evaluative focus should remain on 'the system', particularly at this early developmental stage. After all, the organisational functioning and performance of the revalidation system as a quality assurance tool is, in these risk-aware times, one of medicine's "'visible markers" of trust [which as] … tools of bureaucratic regulation fulfil [a] function as signifiers of quality' (Kuhlmann 2006: 617).

Hence, it is perhaps not so important to ask: 'What are doctors' experiences and opinions of revalidation?', but rather the following key questions:

- How many underperforming doctors is revalidation identifying?
- How does its processes and outcomes link to NHS systems of good clinical governance as well as professional mechanisms of practitioner mentoring, training and professional development?
- How does its processes and outcomes link to key regulatory processes such as the GMC's FPP process?

Finding these answers will take substantial time and resource. Indeed, it is arguable that it will take at least a decade – two revalidation cycles – before we have the necessary initial longitudinal system process and outcome data, from which to form an accurate judgement on system success in protecting the public from harm.

Medical revalidation is undoubtedly a complex intervention that is taking place within an even more complex system of healthcare delivery. But at an organisational and institutional systemic level there are two aspects of revalidation that need to be examined:

- At the local level, there is the provision of CPD opportunities, resources and training for appraisees as well as the selection, training and ongoing quality assurance of the RO, alongside the nature of the local clinical governance and professional practice quality assurance systems in place to respond to appraisal and revalidation outcomes.
- At the national training and regulatory level, the GMC and the professional associations – for example the Royal Colleges – are involved in implementing, supporting and overseeing revalidation processes and outcomes.

When revalidation was implemented nationally in 2012, there were 252,553 doctors on the medical register (GMC 2013c). Latest 2015 figures show that 103,070 doctors have been subject to revalidation: of these, 84,032 have been revalidated, 18,911 were deferred, and there were 127 non-engagements, while a further 1,081 have voluntarily relinquished their licence to practise (GMC 2015). Of the 127 approved non-engagement recommendations, the following outcomes apply: licence withdrawn 28; no longer licensed / registered 37; in the process of licence withdrawal (includes appeals within FPP process) 48; and continues to hold a licence 14.

In relation to deferrals, ROs can recommend a deferral for two reasons: insufficient evidence on which to base a recommendation; or an ongoing local process that needs to be concluded before a recommendation is made. The former can be for a range of reasons, for example a doctor is still completing training in order to enter the medical register, or is taking (or has recently taken) a career break, while the latter typically involves a doctor being subject to local disciplinary or national FPP processes. Indeed, key emergent statistical trends in relation to deferrals include that trainees are more likely to defer while they wait for their training period to finish and acquire their certification of completion of training and for there to be a substantially higher deferral rate of women in their thirties taking career breaks to raise families than for other age groups and genders. There is also some emerging anecdotal evidence that overseas and minority ethnic doctors are more likely to defer or voluntarily relinquish their licences. Furthermore, a recent survey for the GMC, geared to gauging perceptions of fairness for minority ethnic doctors and non-UK graduates, found that only half of respondents thought that revalidation would have any value for patient safety (National Centre for Social Research 2014).

Currently, the GMC has appointed a UK-wide collaboration of researchers entitled UMbRELLA (Uk Medical Revalidation Evaluation coLLAboration), to carry out an independent long-term evaluation of revalidation. It will publish its final report in 2018 – two years after revalidation has been fully implemented nationally and six years after the first doctor was revalidated in 2012. As already noted, it is arguable that the developing dataset and trends therein need to be critically investigated in such a way that we obtain a fully 'joined-up' evaluation of the impact of revalidation. In this age of big data it is no longer acceptable for risk-based governance systems to operate in relative practical and statistical isolation. This is particularly the case when the goal is to identify and address poor medical practice within the NHS in order to minimise the potential for harm to the public and improve patient treatment and care. As well as that, it is widely perceived within the medical profession that Harold Shipman would have been revalidated with ease (Dalrymple 2011). If we are to judge the long-term impact of current reforms in the performance management and quality assurance of medical work, we need to make sure that we have the right analytical tools and data sources at our disposal. It remains to be seen whether current provision will prove to be adequate in this regard.

References

Allsop, J and Mulcahy, L (1996) *Regulating Medical Work: Formal and Informal Controls* (Milton Keynes: Open University Press)

Berg, M (1997) Problems and Promises of the Protocol, *Social Science and Medicine*, 44: 1081-8

Brennan, N, Bryce, M, Pearson, M, Wong, G, Cooper, C and Archer, J (2014) Understanding How Appraisal of Doctors Produces its Effects: A Realist Review Protocol, *BMJ Open*, 4: 54-66

British Medical Association (BMA) (2015) *Revalidation* (London: BMA)

Catto, G (2006) *GMC News 3* (London: GMC)

Catto, G (2007) Will We Be Getting Good Doctors and Safer Patients?, *BMJ*, 334: 450

Chamberlain, J M (2009) Portfolio-based Performance Appraisal for Doctors: A Case of Paperwork Compliance, *Sociological Research Online*, 15, www.socresonline.org.uk/15/1/8.html

Chamberlain, J M (2010) *Doctoring Medical Governance: Medical Regulation in Transition* (NY: Nova Science Publishers)

Chamberlain, J M (2012) *The Sociology of Medical Regulation: An Introduction* (London: Springer)

Checkland, K, McDonald, R and Harrison, S (2007) Ticking Boxes and Changing the Social World: Data Collection and the New UK General Practice Contract, *Social Policy and Administration*, 41: 693-710

Coburn, D and Willis, E (2000) The Medical Profession: Knowledge, Power and Autonomy, in Albrecht, G L, Fitzpatrick, R and Scrimshaw, S C (eds) *The Handbook of Social Science and Medicine* (London: Sage Publications)

Dalrymple, T (2011) Dr Shipman's Review Copy, *BMJ*, 343: 46

Department of Health (DOH) (1989) *Working for Patients* (London: DOH)

DOH (1991) *The Patient's Charter* (London: DOH)

DOH (1999) *Supporting Doctors, Protecting Patients* (London: DOH)

DOH (2000) *The NHS Plan* (London: DOH)

DOH (2014) *Guidance on the Role of Responsible Officer* (London: DOH)

Donaldson, L (2006) *Good Doctors, Safer Patients: Proposals to Strengthen the System to Assure and Improve the Performance of Doctors and to Protect the Safety of Patients* (London: DOH)

Finlay, K and McLaren, S (2009) Does Appraisal Enhance Learning, Improve Practice and Encourage Continuing Professional Development? A Survey of General Practitioners' Experiences of Appraisal, *Quality in Primary Care*, 17: 387-95

Fletcher, C (1997) *Appraisal: Routes to Improved Performance* (London: Short Run Press)

Flynn, R (1992) *Structures of Control in Health Management* (London: Routledge)

Foucault, M (1991) Governmentality, in Burchell, G, Gordon, C and Miller, P (eds) *The Foucault Effect: Studies in Governmentality* (London: Harvester Wheatsheaf)

Freidson, E (2001) *Professionalism: The Third Logic* (Cambridge: Polity Press)

General Medical Council (GMC) (1995) *Duties of a Doctor* (London: GMC)

GMC (1999) *Report of the Revalidation Steering Group* (London: GMC)

GMC (2000) *Revalidating Doctors: Ensuring Standards, Securing the Future* (London: GMC)

GMC (2012) *Ready for Revalidation: Supporting Information for Appraisal and Revalidation* (London: GMC)

GMC (2013a) *Good Medical Practice* (London: GMC)

GMC (2013b) *Revalidation: What You Need to Do* (London: GMC)

GMC (2013c) *The State of Medical Regulation and Medical Education: A Report* (London: GMC)

GMC (2014) *The Good Medical Practice Framework for Appraisal and Revalidation* (London: GMC)

GMC (2015) *Revalidation Implementation Advisory Board – Progress Report March 2015* (London: GMC)

Gentleman, D (2001) The Changing Face of Medical Regulation in the UK, *Clinical Risk*, 7: 169-75

Gladstone, D (2000) *Regulating Doctors* (London: Institute for the Study of Civil Society)

Harrison, S and Schultz, R L (1989) Clinical Autonomy in the UK and the USA: Contrasts and Convergence, in Freddi, G and Bjorkman, J W (eds) *Controlling Medical Professionals: The Comparative Politics of Health Governance* (London: Sage Publications)

Hopkins, A (1990) *Measuring Quality of Medical Care* (London: Royal College of Physicians)

Irvine, D (2003) *The Doctors' Tale: Professionalism and the Public Trust* (London: Radcliffe Medical Press)

Kennedy, I (1983) *The Unmasking of Medicine: A Searching Look at Health Care Today* (London: Granada Publishing)

King's Fund (2014) Kings Fund (2014) *Revalidation: From Compliance to Commitment* London: Kings Fund

Kuhlmann, E (2006) Traces of Doubt and Sources of Trust: Health Professions in an Uncertain Society, *Current Sociology*, 54: 607-19

Lloyd-Bostock, S and Hutter, B (2008) Reforming Regulation of the Medical Profession: The Risks of Risk Based Approaches, *Health, Risk and Society*, 10: 69-83

McDonald, R, Harrison, S, Checkland, K (2008) Incentives and Control in Primary Health Care: Findings from English Pay-for-Performance Case Studies, *Journal of Health Organisation and Management*, 22: 48-62

Mugweni, K, Kibble, S and Conlon, M (2011) Benefits of Appraisal as Perceived by General Practitioners, *Education for Primary Care*, 22: 393-8

National Centre for Social Research (2014) *Fairness and the GMC: Doctors' Views* (London: NCSR)

Newton, T and Findlay, P (1996) Playing God? The Performance of Appraisal, *Human Resource Management*, 6: 42-58

NHS Executive (1994) *Risk Management in the NHS* (Leeds: NHSE)

NHS Revalidation Support Team (2014) *The Early Benefits and Impact of Medical Revalidation: Report on Research Findings in Year One* (London: DOH)

Overeem, K, Faber, M J, Arah, O A, Elwyn, G, Lombarts, K M J M H, Wollersheim, H C (2007) Doctor Performance Assessment in Daily Practice: Does it Help Doctors or Not? A Systematic Review, *Medical Education*, 41: 1039-49

Pollitt, C (1993) Audit and Accountability: The Missing Dimension?, *Journal of the Royal Society of Medicine*, 86: 209-11

Power, M (2007) *Organized Uncertainty: Designing a World of Risk Management* (Oxford: Oxford University Press)

Pym, D. (1973) The Politics and Ritual of Appraisal *Occupational Psychology* (47): 231-35

Redman (1995) Redman, W. (1995 second edition) *Portfolios for Development: a Guide for Trainers and Managers* (London: Kogan Page)

Redman, T, Snape, E, Thompson, D and Ka-Ching, F Y (2000) Performance Appraisal in an NHS hospital, *Human Resource Management Journal*, 10: 48-62

Rose, N (2000) *Powers of Freedom: Reframing Political Thought* (Cambridge: Cambridge University Press)

Sheaff, R, Rogers, A, Pickard, S, Marshall, M, Campbell, S, Sibbald, B, Halliwell, S and Roland, M (2003) A Subtle Governance: 'Soft' Medical Leadership in English Primary Care, *Sociology of Health and Illness*, 25: 408-28

Smith, J (2005) *Shipman: Final Report* (London: DOH)

Smith, R (1992) The GMC on Performance: Professional Self-Regulation is On The Line, *BMJ*, 304: 1257

Smith, R (1998) All Changed, Changed Utterly, *BMJ*, 316: 1917-18

Smither, J W and London, M (2009) *Performance Management: Putting Research into Action* (London: John Wiley & Sons)

Snadden, D and Thomas, M (1998) The Use of Portfolio Learning in Medical Education, *Medical Teacher*, 20: 244-65

Southgate, L (2001) The General Medical Council's Performance Procedures: Study of the Implementation and Impact, *Medical Education*, 35: 23-45

Townley, B (1993a) Foucault, Power/Knowledge, and its Relevance for Human Resource Management, *Academy of Management Review*, 18: 518-45

Townley, B (1993b) Performance Appraisal and the Emergence of Human Resource Management, *Journal of Management Studies*, 30: 221-38

Townley, B (1999) Practical Reason and Performance Appraisal, *Journal of Management Studies*, 36: 287-306

Wennberg, J (1988) Practice Variations and the Need for Outcomes Research, in Ham, C (ed.) *Health Care Variations: Assessing the Evidence* (London: King's Fund Institute)

West, M A, Borrill, C, Dawson, J, Scully, J, Carter, M, Anelay, S et al (2002) The Link Between the Management of Employees and Patient Mortality in Acute Hospitals, *International Journal of Human Resource Management*, 13: 1299-310

Wilkinson, T J, Challis, M, Hobma, S O, Newble, D I, Parbossingh, J T, Sibbald, R G and Wakefield, R (2002) The Use of Portfolios for Assessment of the Competence and Performance of Doctors in Practice, *Medical Education*, 36: 23-46

Zuboff, S (1988) *In the Age of the Smart Machine* (Oxford: Heinemann)

FITNESS TO PRACTISE PANELS: THE MEDICAL PRACTITIONERS TRIBUNAL SERVICE

Introduction

The previous chapter provided a critical introduction into the development, implementation and evaluation of medical revalidation as a system of governance designed to ensure that practitioners remain up to date and fit to practise in their chosen specialty. In this chapter, we look more closely at the processes in place for when a complaint is made against a doctor and their fitness to practise is called into question.

As already noted, the medical register of approved practitioners is overseen by the GMC under the aegis of the Medical Act 1983. The GMC is, therefore, the statutory body responsible for responding to complaints about the fitness to practise of doctors and has the authority to remove them from the register by instigating disciplinary proceedings via a fitness to practise panel (FPP). In 2014, the Law Commission's comprehensive review of healthcare professionals (2014a) noted that medical FPPs are a vitally important legal mechanism for ensuring that public trust in medical regulation is maintained when complaints are made about a doctor and, as a result, it has acted to strengthen the investigatory and adjudication process, by legislating to ensure that the panels are independent, autonomous structures of the GMC.

Official figures show that when revalidation was implemented nationally in 2012, there were 252,553 doctors on the medical register, and in 2012 a complaint was registered against 4% (10,347) of doctors and less than 1% (208) were removed from the medical register (GMC 2013). This is a very small proportion of practising doctors in the UK. Nevertheless, as this chapter will outline, year on year over the last decade the number of complaints made to the GMC has increased. Moreover, the rise in the volume of complaints has been accompanied by a growing perception within the medical profession that the GMC itself is far less tolerant of infractions than before.

After the respective Bristol and Shipman cases, there was broad consensus within the medical profession that substantive changes were needed to reform both the organisation and working culture of the GMC, to ensure that underperforming doctors, as well as those engaging in malpractice and/or acts of criminality, could be more easily prevented from continuing to practise. Under the Health and Social Care Act 2008, the standard of evidence required to secure a guilty verdict and to remove a practitioner from the medical register was reduced from a criminal standard of proof to a civil standard of proof. This change was justified on the grounds that, historically, the GMC had often been unable to remove a doctor from the medical register, even when doubt existed over their clinical performance, because the standard of proof required was unduly high and significantly affected the number of successful prosecutions.

However, legislative reform is associated with a wider political agenda, buttressed by media coverage of high-profile medical error cases, such as Mid-Staffordshire NHS Trust, which seeks to minimise clinical risk and cost through the transformation of medical work into a series of routine 'step-by-step' rules and procedures, against which individual clinician performance can be measured and judged. The concern here is that legal reforms have been introduced to the FPP process for reasons that fail to fully account for the nature of medical discretion and, as a result, they may unintentionally serve, in particular types of cases, to undermine the principles of swift, proportionate and effective legal response(s) to ensure public protection.

This proposition is particularly prescient in light of the highly politicised nature of the legal regulation of doctors more generally, and given that the patient complaint system (out of necessity) provides a reactive, service user-led mechanism of professional accountability, in which notions of due process, fairness and redress must be carefully balanced. Against the backdrop of these recent legislative reforms in medical regulation and current parliamentary debates pertaining to changes in FPPs proposed by the Law Commission, this chapter examines the operation of the GMC complaints procedure and provides an analysis of statistical trends over time in the outcomes of FPPs. A key part of this is the examination of the impact (if any) of the shift in the standard of evidence required under the 'realistic prospect test' to remove a doctor from the medical register.

The chapter argues that the handling of enquiries by the GMC provides a basis on which to analyse its administrative operational procedures in order to identify if, and how far, a cultural change in the organisation has occurred over the last decade since the Shipman report (Smith 2005). It is argued that the statistical data outlined confirms that focusing longitudinally on the management of enquiries and FPP outcomes is an invaluable tool for assessing the impact of regulatory reform on the day-to-day operation of the GMC. Furthermore, it is asserted that the statistical data outlined in this chapter provides evidence for the viewpoint that there has indeed been a change in the operational culture of the GMC, as it is increasingly acting informally to provide advice, to give warnings and to agree rehabilitative forms of action with doctors, as well as more formally to subject doctors to rehabilitative and disciplinary action.

Nevertheless, it is also noted that the shift in the level of evidence required to meet the 'realistic prospect test' does not seem to have resulted in significantly more doctors being struck off the medical register. Furthermore, it is noted that comparing the year-on-year statistical data reveals that even though the number of enquiries has risen by 688% since 1995, the GMC has nevertheless adopted a relatively consistent administrative approach towards the management of cases in terms of the disposal pathway by which they typically progress. Importantly, these findings are congruent with the view that the organisational change underway within the GMC is underpinned by a growing reliance on formulised 'risk templates' to aid decision-making processes. This further supports the position that there has been a shift towards risk-based regulation.

The chapter ends by considering the impact of this state of affairs on medical practitioners. It outlines that it is vitally important that current reforms to the fitness to practise tribunal process proposed by the Law Commission, which appear to be primarily driven by matters of economic efficiency and practical expediency, do not become overly concerned with 'punishment for punishment's sake' as a consequence of a risk-averse drive towards increased medical accountability and institutional transparency. This concluding point helps to set the scene for Chapter Four, which focuses on the issue of punishment under risk-based forms of medical regulation, given contemporary developments in the implementation of medical revalidation and FPPs.

Handling complaints and hearing fitness to practise cases

Before outlining the statistical outcomes of FPP cases, it is first necessary to provide an overview of how the GMC responds to complaints. The GMC is responsible for removing doctors from the medical register. It does not respond to complaints against NHS systems (although it may respond to complaints against individuals that illustrate system failings). Neither does it arrange for complainants to receive an apology, an explanation of what happened, or provide help and support for compensation claims. The GMC is one of a number of bodies that deal with complaints against medical practitioners. NHS hospital trusts and primary care trusts alongside the National Clinical Assessment Service (as part of the NHS Litigation Authority), the Care Quality Commission and the Parliamentary and Health Service Ombudsman, are all important points of contact for dealing with medical malpractice and patient complaints. But the GMC remains the only body able to remove a doctor from the medical register and, as a result, stop them from practising medicine in the UK.

The GMC only responds to complaints that call into question a doctor's fitness to practise (GMC 2004a). Under section 35C(2) of the Medical Act 1983, alongside the guidance to good practice provided in its document *Good Medical Practice*, the GMC focuses on complaints that highlight instances where a doctor has:

- made serious or repeated mistakes in carrying out medical procedures or in diagnosis (for example by prescribing drugs in a dangerous way);
- not examined a patient properly or responded appropriately to their medical need;
- committed fraud, dishonesty or serious breaches of a patient confidentiality;
- received a criminal conviction;
- developed a physical and/or mental health issue (GMC 2013a).

All complaints made to the GMC are referred to initially as 'enquiries'. The GMC's fitness to practise procedures are divided into two key stages: investigation and adjudication (GMC 2014). The purpose of the investigation stage is to make an assessment as to whether there is a need to refer an enquiry to the Medical Practitioners Tribunal Service (MPTS) for adjudication, which consists of a hearing by an FPP. During the investigative stage, a 'triage' process takes place, which involves making an initial decision as to whether or not to proceed with an enquiry. Some enquiries are clearly outside the GMC's remit. For example, an enquiry may not be concerned with an individual medical practitioner. Enquiries which are clearly outside the GMC's remit and do not enter the investigative stage are referred to as 'stream two' enquiries and are discontinued with no further action. If necessary, the GMC will refer the matter to the doctor's employer, so that local procedures can be used if necessary to respond to it. If the initial information points towards the existence of a criminal conviction, then the matter will be immediately referred to an MPTS FPP for adjudication.

In those instances where the triage process confirms that the enquiry requires further consideration, the GMC will proceed to the investigative stage. At this point, the GMC will disclose the complaint to the doctor in question as well as their employer, to ensure that a complete picture of their practice can be obtained. All cases are overseen by two 'case examiners', one of whom is a non-medical practitioner and one a medical practitioner. Witness statements and supportive material will be collected and analysed, including copies of patient medical records or other formal documentary material (for example, employer reports).

Where there is a concern with performance or health, appropriate tests will be completed at this stage and an interim orders panel may be held. This panel may decide to suspend or restrict a doctor's practice while the investigation continues. The investigation period concludes with either no further action being taken, the issuing of a warning, a practitioner agreeing to what are referred to as 'undertakings', or a case being referred to an MPTS FPP for adjudication. In 2013, the majority of enquiries took 29 weeks to move from the initial complaint to investigation outcome stage (PSA 2014).

The adjudication stage involves a formal hearing of a case by an MPTS FPP. The panel is made up of medical and non-medical lay members. The format is adversarial, with the GMC's legal representative presenting evidence and argument in the public interest, and a practitioner's legal representative similarly presenting their own argument and evidence. If necessary, the panel will be advised by a specialist health and/or performance adviser.

There are five main outcomes of a FPP meeting:

- no further action;
- issuing a doctor with a formal warning;
- placing restrictions on a doctor's professional practice (for example, imposing supervision or requiring the doctor to undertake further training);

- suspending a doctor from the medical register so that they may not practise for a given period of time;
- erasing a doctor from the medical register.

It is the intention of the GMC when they erase a doctor from the medical register that this ought normally to be for life. In 2013, most enquiries took 97 weeks to move from the initial complaint to MPTS FPP outcome stage (PSA 2014).

A doctor has 28 days to appeal against a decision, which they lodge at the High Court or the Court of Session. The panel's decision will not take effect until either the appeal period expires or the appeal is determined. However, the panel can impose an immediate order of suspension or conditions on practice, if it believes that this is necessary to protect the public or is in the best interests of the doctor. Furthermore, since 2005 the PSA has the power under section 29 of the National Health Service Reform and Health Care Professions Act 2002 to refer a decision by an MPTS FPP to the High Court (or its equivalent throughout the UK) for the protection of the public, if it considers a decision to be unduly lenient. The PSA has 28 days to decide whether to refer a decision following the doctor's 28-day appeal period. In 2013-14, it did so on three occasions (PSA 2014).

Additionally, the PSA reviews all decisions of MPTS FPPs that have not resulted in erasure from the medical register. It forwarded four such cases in 2005, six in 2006, none in 2007, one in 2008, one in 2009, two in 2010, one in 2011, none in 2012 and none in 2013 (CHRE 2005, 2006, 2007, 2008, 2009, 2010, 2011; PSA 2013, 2014). The small number of referrals might suggest an increasingly rigorous stance on behalf of the GMC towards fitness to practise cases, at least since it became subject to regulatory oversight by the PSA. However, to ascertain whether this is the case, it is necessary to examine the operation over time of the GMC's investigatory and adjudication process.

Trends in the GMC investigatory and adjudication procedures

This section details the main features of enquiry data obtained from the GMC for the period between 2006 and 2012, with data from previous years being discussed where possible. Contact was made with the GMC to discuss the availability of data, under the Freedom of Information Act 2000. It was stated by the GMC that they have only held fully computerised record systems since 2006 and that the resources that would need to be allocated to review stored paper files to obtain data prior to this date would exceed the appropriate limit of costs incurred. This has been set at £450 for public authorities under the Freedom of Information and Data Protection (Appropriate Limit and Fees) Regulations 2004.

The GMC noted that it was possible to obtain data on complaints for 1995, 1998 and between 1999 and 2012, as well as the hearing of fitness to practise cases for the years 2006 to 2012, from a range of published reports.[8] Before outlining the data, it is important to note that although it descriptively illustrates the operation of the GMC, it should not be taken as representative of its total activity for each calendar year. As already noted, in 2013 an enquiry took on average 97 weeks to move from the initial complaint to MPTS FPP outcome stage. Hence an enquiry received in 2009 may well not reach resolution until 2011. That said, having year-on-year comparative data does allow for descriptive statistical trends to emerge, as the next section will illustrate.

Number of enquiries and their source

The total number of enquiries received by the GMC between 1999 and 2012 are detailed in Table 1. This table also shows the number of enquiries received by the GMC in 1995 and in 1998. The figures for 1995 and 1998 were obtained from the aforementioned published GMC documents. Aside from 2006, when the number of enquiries reduced sharply, the figures reveal that the number of enquiries received by the GMC has increased by 688% in the 17 years between 1995 and 2012: from 1,503 in 1995 to 10,347 in 2012. The total of 10,347 enquiries represents 4% of all medical practitioners on the GMC register (252,553) (GMC 2013b). Although the GMC did change to a fully computerised record system in 2006, the dip in enquiries that year cannot be attributed to any major change in the organisation or role of the GMC, so it may well be simply a statistical aberration, which can routinely occur in the analysis of longitudinal data. Furthermore, its presence does little to alter the significance of the longitudinal trend for increased enquiries.

It appears that enquiries doubled between the mid and late 1990s, with the number trebling into the beginning of the new millennium, before evening off slightly (aside from in 2006) until increasing back up again year on year since 2009. This trend provides empirical evidence for the argument that in the last two decades there has been an *increase* in the questioning of medical authority, with the result that individuals are more likely to complain about their doctor and/or the treatment they have received (Archer 2014). Moreover, it is likely that high-profile medical malpractice cases, such as the respective Bristol and Shipman cases for example, have significantly raised the profile of the GMC in the media and with the general public, resulting in a dramatic increase in the number of enquiries that the GMC receives.

In order to critically examine the validity of this possible correlation, it is necessary to identify the source of enquiries. Table 2 illustrates that while the majority of enquiries received originate from the general public, there has been a gradual

Table 1: Number of complaints received by the GMC (1995–2012)

Year	Number of enquiries
2012	10,347
2011	8,781
2010	7,153
2009	5,773
2008	4,166
2007	4,118
2006	2,788
2005	4,128
2004	4,005
2003	3,962
2002	3,937
2001	4,504
2000	4,470
1999	3,001
1998	3,066
1995	1,503

increase in enquiries from other sources in recent years, which most typically include employers, other doctors, other health and social care professionals, as well as the police. This is congruent with the more proactive stance that the GMC is taking towards working with local NHS employers and private healthcare providers as it seeks to promote a working culture that encourages complainants to present their concerns without fearing negative consequences for their career. This has historically been recognised as a key issue affecting a potential complainant's willingness to instigate proceedings/present their concerns (GMC 2013b).

Table 2: Source of enquiry (1995-2012)

Year	Percentage of enquiries from the public	Percentage of enquiries from other sources
2012	62	38
2011	65	35
2010	63	37
2009	64	36
2008	68	32
2007	70	30
2006	66	34
2005	73	27
2004	74	26
2003	77	23
2002	76	24
2001	75	25
2000	73	27
1999	Data not available	Data not available
1998	Data not available	Data not available
1995	Data not available	Data not available

Investigatory stage outcomes

Having examined the number of enquiries made, it is now necessary to consider the figures relating to the progression of cases from the investigation and adjudication stages. It was impossible to identify comparative outcome figures for the handling of enquiries at the investigative and adjudication stages prior to 2006 from the reports available, as the process by which the GMC handles enquiries changed at this time as a consequence of broader reforms introduced following the Shipman case. Nevertheless, the available data for 2006 to 2012 can be compared and reveals several key trends in the GMC case management of enquiries. First, it is important to review what occurred after each enquiry was received by the GMC, displayed in Table 3.

Table 3: Enquiries received and concluded (2006-2012)

Year	Received	Concluded	% concluded
2012	10,347	7,639	74
2011	8,781	6,451	74
2010	7,153	5,087	72
2009	5,773	4,015	70
2008	4,166	3,530	85
2007	4,118	3,722	90
2006	2,788	2,442	88

Table 3 reveals important year-on-year consistencies in the GMC handling of enquiries received and subsequent actions undertaken , with between two-thirds and four-fifths of cases being concluded at the initial complaint stage.

Moreover, in view of the time taken for a case to reach completion, GMC outcomes generally tend to roll forward to the following reporting period. Although there has been an increase in the number of enquiries received and an increase in the number of enquiries proceeding to investigation (from 12% in 2006 when the GMC was reformed, to 26% in 2012), over the last four years (2008-12) around three-quarters of enquiries have resulted in no action being taken against a doctor. In short, it does not necessarily follow that the increase in enquiries has resulted in significantly more doctors being formally investigated by the GMC.

Indeed, Table 4, which details the outcomes when investigatory action has occurred, reveals that an initial increase between 2006 and 2008 in warnings and rehabilitative undertakings, as well as a trend for more cases being referred to the MPTS FPP, gave way between 2010 and 2012 to an increase in the GMC providing individuals (and their employers) with informal advice and guidance, and in fact, the number of FPP referrals has subsequently reduced.

Table 4: Breakdown of GMC investigatory action outcomes (2006-2012)

Year	Action: advice	Action: warning issued	Action: undertakings	Referred to FPP
2012	844	182	143	216
2011	736	199	148	212
2010	458	183	102	314
2009	428	212	95	319
2008	Not available	168	109	359
2007	Not available	159	40	196
2006	Not available	86	44	216

FPP outcomes

The data included in Tables 1–4 provides evidence on how complaints are managed by the GMC at the initial investigative stage. It is now necessary to detail the outcomes of cases heard at the adjudication stage by an MPTS FPP. This data is found in Table 5.

For year-on-year comparative purposes, the data has been broken down into relative percentages for each action category, based on the total number of cases heard per year. This shows that there is a relatively strong degree of year-on-year consistency in the types of action taken at the adjudication stage. For example, year on year, the proportion of

Table 5: Fitness to practise panel outcomes

Case outcome	2006		2007		2008		2009		2010		2011		2012	
	N=221	100%	N=257	100%	N=204	100%	N=270	100%	N=326	100%	N=242	100%	N=208	100%
Cases heard														
Impairment – no action	8	4%	13	5%	4	2%	4	1%	4	1%	2	1%	6	3%
No Impairment – no action	47	21%	36	14%	28	14%	44	16%	65	20%	33	14%	48	23%
Voluntary Erasure	3	1%	2	1%	0	0%	3	1%	7	2%	1	>0.5%	2	1%
Undertakings	4	2%	4	2%	3	1%	3	1%	5	2%	1	>0.5%	1	>0.5%
Reprimand	1	1%	1	1%	0	0%	1	1%	0	0%	0	0%	0	0%
Warning	14	6%	8	3%	22	11%	22	8%	29	9%	23	10%	12	6%
Conditions	38	17%	55	21%	30	15%	48	18%	37	11%	24	10%	20	10%
Suspension	69	31%	78	30%	75	37%	77	29%	106	33%	93	38%	64	31%
Erasure	37	17%	60	23%	42	20%	68	25%	73	22%	65	27%	55	26%

cases which lead to a doctor being erased from the medical register are: 17% in 2006, 23% in 2007, 20% in 2008, 25% in 2009, 22% in 2010, 27% in 2011 and 26% in 2012. Cases which result in no impairment and no action are: 21% in 2006, 14% in 2007, 14% in 2008, 16% in 2009, 20% in 2010, 14% in 2011 and 23% in 2012.

Although there is a degree of fluctuation in the year-on-year percentages within each case disposal pathway, overall the data demonstrates that there is a strong element of comparative consistency, both between and within the different action categories, in how the GMC managed fitness to practise cases from 2006 to 2012.

Furthermore, this period has been accompanied by a growing public concern about medical error and malpractice, alongside an increasing perception within the medical profession at large that the GMC is adopting a more punitive approach to the management of fitness to practise cases. In this regard, Table 5 reinforces that the adjudication stage is more likely to result in high impact decisions, such as conditions being placed on a doctor's practice, suspension from the medical register or erasure from the medical register.

Relatively few doctors receive undertakings or warnings at adjudication stage, although a considerable percentage of cases result in the conclusion that there is no impairment in a doctor's practice. The most significant observation, however, is that the shift to a civil standard of proof during this time period (that is from 2008 onwards) *does not* appear to have resulted in an immediate and significant increase in doctors being erased from the medical register.

Next steps: the MPTS, FPPs and the Law Commission Review

Although greater numbers of doctors are being subject to informal and formal forms of action by the GMC, the data outlined in this paper conclusively demonstrates that the shift towards a civil standard of proof *has not* led to significantly more doctors being removed from the medical register. This is a pertinent finding, given current developments surrounding the role of the GMC in relation to case investigation and adjudication. The Health and Social Care Act 2008 established the Office of Health Professions Adjudicator (OHPA) to take over the role of the GMC in the adjudication of fitness to practise cases. The intended aim of this change was to enhance impartiality and the independence of the fitness to practise hearing process within the healthcare professions (Department of Health 2009)

The OHPA became a legal entity in January 2010. Yet in the summer of 2010, the UK government concluded that it was not persuaded of the need to introduce another regulatory body to fulfil the role of adjudicator in fitness to practise cases (Department of Health 2010). In part, this decision was made in light of the stringent economic realities faced by public services in the UK as the state sought to respond to the financial realities of the 2008 global financial crisis. The GMC is predominately funded by the medical profession via an annual subscription fee, and there was concern that implementing further reform would potentially result in additional cost to the public purse.

Furthermore, this decision was also a reflection of the extent to which medical elites, notably the Royal Colleges, had successfully persuaded government that they had managed to subject 'rank and file' practitioners to greater peer surveillance and control, albeit under the ever watchful gaze of the state and its regulatory oversight body, the PSA (McGivern and Fischer 2010). However, the research finding that a significant number of enquiries continued to fail to make it past the initial triage and investigative stages has in the intervening period raised questions about the GMC's gatekeeper role at each point in the decision-making and follow-up process. This is not least because the little independent research into the GMC management of complaints that existed in the past revealed the apparent presence of judgemental bias (Allen 2000), and a small-scale independent review of a sample of GMC complaints found that: 'articulate individuals who present their complaints clearly and in detail are more likely to have their cases taken up by the GMC' (Hughes 2007: 15). Similarly, the PSA, when it was called the CHRE, stated, in light of its audit of GMC operations, that: 'We consider that it [the GMC] needs to ensure that its decision makers have fully understood all the complainant's concerns, and that complainants feel that they are encouraged to submit a complaint' (CHRE 2010: 17).

In response to such concerns, the Law Commission began a consultation exercise to reform the FPP process in 2012, in order to establish areas for further regulatory reform, particularly in relation to the GMC responses to enquiries and the FPP process (Law Commission 2014a, 2014b, 2014c). At the same time, the GMC established the MPTS to assume responsibility for the adjudication of FPP cases (GMC 2011b). This is not the first time that the GMC has acted pre-emptively to reform its internal organisation in the face of governmental consultation in relation to reforming its statutory powers. At the centre of the consultation sits the need to address the issue that the GMC is currently responsible for both the investigation and the adjudication of allegations of impaired fitness to practise. As arbiters of standards and prosecutor decision-making, the GMC's independence as adjudicator acting in the interests of the public is arguably tenuous and open to question. That the change in the 'realistic prospect test' has not resulted in more doctors being struck off the medical register does lend some support to the argument that a conflict of interest continues to exist in spite of recent regulatory reform.

Two solutions have been proposed:

- the creation of an independent body to oversee adjudication and for the GMC to be solely concerned with investigation before passing cases on to this body; or
- for the MPTS to be an independent arm of the GMC responsible for adjudication.

In both instances, the PSA will retain regulatory oversight and the right to refer FPP outcomes to the High Court under section 29 of the National Health Service Reform and Health Care Professions Act 2002. As of spring 2015, the current proposals to be laid before Parliament, are for the GMC to establish internal structural mechanisms, which ensure a greater degree of separation, with the

MPTS becoming a clearly distinctive and autonomous arm of the organisation responsible for case adjudication.

There will, therefore, be a separation of the GMC's investigative and adjudicatory roles. Additionally, if these proposals are accepted, the GMC's investigatory arm will have the right to appeal a case decision. It is argued by the Law Commission that the: 'General Medical Council's proposed right of appeal is both a consequence of, and reinforces, the independence of the new Medical Practitioners Tribunal Service' (Law Commission 2014a: 211). It is proposed that under statutory instruments (as yet to be defined), this right of appeal will be used when a sanction is considered to be unduly lenient or, in relation to a decision not to take any disciplinary action or restore a person to the register, that the decision should not have been made.

The original intention behind establishing an 'in house', quasi-independent MPTS within the GMC's organisational structure was to remove the unsatisfactory situation of it acting as 'judge and jury' in fitness to practise cases (Case 2011). It is held to be the most appropriate solution in view of concerns expressed within the medical profession and government, in regard to the utility of adopting alternative (more costly) approaches, given the self-funding nature of the GMC and the highly specialised nature of medical expertise (GMC 2013c). Furthermore, the decision to embed within statutory legislation the right of the GMC to appeal MPTS decisions to the High Court, in addition to the right of the PSA to appeal decisions in a similar fashion, adds a 'double layer' of regulatory oversight to FPP outcomes process, and reflects the emphasis placed by risk-averse regulatory models on minimising the possibility of harm.

Nonetheless, embedding the MPTS within the GMC, rather than an independent body such as the (now defunct) OHPA, suggests that matters of economic efficiency and practical expediency have taken precedence over public interest. Additionally, it is equally important to consider the language in use here within the context of matters of due process. Doctors who are subject to MPTS proceedings have the right to expect a fair hearing. Focusing on legislating for the right of regulatory bodies to appeal decisions made in tribunal as a result of the adversarial process, is arguably indicative of a process that is becoming overly politicised and unduly weighted towards the pursuit of punishment, rather than retaining a necessary emphasis on balancing notions of fairness with redress (McCartney 2014)

Conclusion

The data presented in this paper conclusively demonstrates that the shift in the level of evidence required to meet the 'realistic prospect test' has not resulted in significantly more doctors being struck off the medical register, while the FPP outcome suspension and erasure pathways have remained relatively static over the reporting period. The chapter situated these findings within the context of current legal regulatory consultations underway to further reform the FPP process by embedding an MPTS as a separate arm within the GMC. This consultation is designed to ensure the heightened visibility of dangerous doctors and to ameliorate responses to instances of medical malpractice and criminality.

However, under the proposed recommendations, two regulatory bodies – the GMC and its oversight body the PSA – will be able to appeal decisions made in tribunal. This raises the possibility that the process may become unduly weighted towards the pursuit of punishment, rather than retaining a necessary emphasis on balancing notions of fairness with redress.

In the next chapter, this discussion is brought together with that in the previous chapter concerned with medical revalidation, to highlight that current legal regulatory effort to promote trust in medical regulation must not allow the concomitant shift towards risk-averse forms of professional accountability to sacrifice public safety and due legal process for the sake of political pragmatic exigency.

References

Allen, I (2000) *The Handling of Complaints by the GMC: A Study of Decision Making and Outcomes* (London: Policy Studies Institute)

Archer, J (2014) *Understanding the Rise in Fitness to Practice Complaints from the Public* (Plymouth: Plymouth Medical School)

Case, P (2011) The Good, the Bad and the Dishonest Doctor: the General Medical Council and the Redemption Model of Fitness to Practice, *Legal Studies*, 31: 591-614

Council for Healthcare Regulatory Excellence (CHRE) (2005) *Statistical Summary 2005* (London: CHRE)

CHRE (2006) *Statistical Summary 2006* (London: CHRE)

CHRE (2007) *Statistical Summary 2007* (London: CHRE)

CHRE (2008) *Statistical Summary 2008* (London: CHRE)

CHRE (2009) *Statistical Summary 2009* (London: CHRE)

CHRE (2010) *Statistical Summary 2010* (London: CHRE)

CHRE (2011) *Statistical Summary 2011* (London: CHRE)

Department of Health (2009) *Health Care Regulation: Tackling Concerns Nationally* (London: DOH)

Department of Health (2010) *Fitness to Practice Adjudication for Health Professionals* (London: DOH)

General Medical Council (GMC) (2000) *Annual Statistics* (London: GMC)

GMC (2001) *Annual Statistics* (London: GMC)

GMC (2002) *Annual Statistics* (London: GMC)

GMC (2003) *Annual Statistics* (London: GMC)

GMC (2004a) *Guidance on GMC's Fitness to Practise Rule* (London: GMC)

GMC (2004b) *Annual Statistics* (London: GMC)

GMC (2005) *Annual Statistics* (London: GMC)

GMC (2006) *Fitness to Practise: Annual Statistics* (London: GMC)

GMC (2007) *Fitness to Practise: Annual Statistics* (London: GMC)

GMC (2008) *Fitness to Practise: Annual Statistics* (London: GMC)

GMC (2009) *Fitness to Practise: Annual Statistics* (London: GMC)

GMC (2010) *Fitness to Practise: Annual Statistics* (London: GMC)

GMC (2011a) *Fitness to Practise: Annual Statistics* (London: GMC)

GMC (2011b) *The Future of Adjudication and the Establishment of the Medical Practitioners Tribunal Service* (London: GMC)

GMC (2012) *Fitness to Practise: Annual Statistics* (London: GMC)

GMC (2013a) *Good Medical Practice* (London: GMC)

GMC (2013b) *The State of Medical Regulation and Medical Education: A Report* (London: GMC)

GMC (2013c) *Our Response to the Report of the Mid-Staffordshire NHS Foundation Trust Public Inquiry* (London: GMC)

GMC (2014) *Fitness to Practice Procedures* (London: GMC)

Hughes, J (2007) *An Independent Audit of Decisions in the Investigation Stage of the GMC's Fitness to Practice process* (London: King's College London)

Law Commission (2014a) *Regulation of Health Care Professionals, Regulation of Social Care Professionals in England*, Law Commission Consultation Paper No 202 (London Law Commission)

Law Commission (2014b) *Regulation of Health Care Professionals, Regulation of Social Care Professionals in Northern Ireland*, Law Commission Consultation Paper No 12 (Belfast Law Commission)

Law Commission (2014c) *Regulation of Health Care Professionals, Regulation of Social Care Professionals in Scotland* Scottish Law Commission Discussion Paper No 153 (Edinburgh Law Commission)

McCartney, M (2014) Does the GMC Deserve its Current Powers?, *BMJ*, 349: 36-8

McGivern, G and Fischer, M (2010) Medical Regulation, Spectacular Transparency and the Blame Business, *Journal of Health Organisation and Management*, 24: 597-610

Professional Standards Authority (PSA) (2013) *Performance Review Report 2012-13* (London: PSA)

PSA (2014) *Performance Review Report 2013-14* (London: PSA)

Smith, J (2005) *Shipman: Final Report* (London: DOH)

REGULATING FOR THE SAFER DOCTOR IN THE RISK SOCIETY: IS THE PROCESS THE PUNISHMENT?

Introduction

Chapter Two critically explored the introduction of medical revalidation as a regulatory quality assurance measure for ensuring that a medical practitioner remains up to date and fit to practise in their chosen specialty. Chapter Three extended this analysis to the examination of reforms to the tribunal system in place for the hearing of cases when a medical practitioner's fitness to practise has been called into question. These legislative reforms in the regulation of doctors have supported the development of a risk-based model of professional governance, which has prompted fundamental changes in the internal organisational structure of the GMC (Scrivens 2007). The GMC is undoubtedly a very different organisation from what it was previously. No longer is it *the* symbol of medical authority, status and power: the traditional, doctors-only 'club mentality' has shifted to permit the inclusion of non-medical members (Hutter and Power 2005). Consequently, the GMC now possesses open and transparent administrative protocols, processes and outcome measures, from which its operational performance can be independently measured and judged.

In the past, as a result of high-profile scandals, the GMC has been accused of bias towards doctors and has been criticised for not fulfilling its statutory obligation to protect the public. As a result, it has sought to become more transparent in its operations (Waring and Dixon-Woods 2010). In this context, the concept of 'transparency' can be understood as a policy device designed to enable practices that are open to public scrutiny in order to generate greater trust and legitimacy. Furthermore, the introduction of medical revalidation and reforms in the hearing of fitness to practise cases are demonstrative of an organisation undergoing a transition from a reactive, incident-led institution, which has been preoccupied with ensuring medical privilege, to a proactive overseer of professional standards designed to secure the public interest. These developments arguably therefore lend support to the argument often made by political and medical elites that the shift from 'self-regulation' to 'regulated self-regulation' better protects the public interest (Chamberlain 2012).

This chapter reflects on this conclusion in the context of the emergence of the complex media-saturated social conditions associated with the rise of the 'risk society', and examines patient and doctor dissatisfaction with revalidation and the fitness to practise panel (FPP) process through consideration of notions of procedural fairness and justice (Giddens 1999, Beck and Beck-Gernsheim 2002, Power 2007). Risk-averse models of professional regulation rely on codified performance appraisal frameworks to support institutional transparency and generate greater trust in organisational operational procedures (Glynne and Gomez 2005). This state of affairs might not be easily reconcilable with traditional notions of medical collegiality and discretion (Hood 2002).

In the last three decades, the implementation of rule-based structures across public administration in the health and social welfare context has proliferated widely due to the emergence of New Public Management as a reforming driver within the public sphere. This suggests that Dworkin's notions of official, strong and weak forms of discretion (introduced in Chapter One) remain salient in contemporary discussions of professional discretion (Dent et al 2004). Certainly, strong discretion remains *the* defining feature of the practices of both doctors and professional bureaucracies. The movement away from the *Bolam test* standard by virtue of the *Bolitho gloss*, and towards the use of more extrinsic forms of evidence (such as best-evidenced clinical guidelines) to define what constitutes the grounds for decision making in relation to instances of questionable medical practice, has nevertheless recognised that collegiate peer review remains, in the majority of cases, the most appropriate evidential source on which to base case judgement (Havighurst 1991).

Moreover, it is tenuous to assume that placing a legislative regulatory emphasis on promoting institutional transparency will necessarily result in the de facto outcomes intended by government. The presence of 'game playing' by doctors in relation to the use of portfolio-based performance appraisal tools such as annual appraisal, as outlined in Chapter Two, suggests that placing a regulatory emphasis on the promotion of organisational transparency may in fact engender subtle, nuanced or perverse consequences, which act to subvert the public interest and challenge legal notions of fairness (Power 2007).

The rest of Chapter Four explores this issue, while asking the question: 'Under the conditions of the risk society, has the process become the punishment?' To answer this, it is first necessary to document the nature of the patient–public relationship under the social conditions associated with the emerging risk society, as conceptualised by its key advocates.

The rise of the risk society

For many social scientists the re-emergence of liberalism from the 1980s onwards, which was touched on in Chapter Two, coincided with a general social shift towards the conditions of late or high modernity. We certainly live in an increasingly interconnected, technologically advanced world, where events and happenings occurring on the other side of the globe are immediately available for personal consumption (and arguably therefore immediately impact on the sociocultural and economic-political spheres). For social theorists such as Beck (1992) and Giddens (1990, 1991, 1999), a key defining feature of modern society – or 'late' or 'high modernity' as they call it – is that there has been: 'a social impetus towards individualisation of unprecedented scale and dynamism … [which] forces people – for the sake of their survival – to make themselves the centre of their own life plans and conduct' (Beck and Beck-Gernsheim 2002: 31). Both Beck and Giddens argue that as a capitalist-industrial society gives way under the tripartite forces of technology, consumerism and globalisation, there is a categorical shift in the nature of social structures and, more importantly, in the relationship between the individual and society.

Here key sociological categories that have traditionally structured society increasingly lose their meaning. Hence social categories such as race, gender and class, for example, increasingly no longer serve to restrict a person's social opportunities or define who they are as individuals to the extent that they once did. Furthermore, as working conditions change, and the technology and communication revolutions continue apace, more than ever before individuals are required to make life-changing decisions concerning education, work, self-identify and personal relationships, in a world where traditional beliefs about social class, gender and the family are being overturned.

Now for many social theorists this state of affairs has led to a concern with dangerousness and risk entering centre stage within society's institutional governing apparatus, alongside an individual subject-citizen's personal decision-making process (Mythen 2004). As one of the key risk theorists, Giddens (1990) talks about two forms of risk: external and manufactured risk. Put simply, external risks are those posed by the world around us, and manufactured risks are created by human beings themselves. In essence, as Giddens explains, it is the difference between worrying about what nature can do with us – in the form of floods, famine and so on – and worrying about what we have done to the natural world via how we organise social life. But of course it is not that simple. Risk theorists argue that throughout human history, societies have always sought to risk-manage threats, hazards and dangers. But these management activities have, by and large, been concerned with natural external risks, such as infectious diseases and famine.

However, in today's technologically advanced society, individuals are seen to be both the producers and minimisers of manufactured risk (Giddens 1990). That is, within the conditions of high modernity, risks are seen to be solely the result of human activity (Mythen 2004). Hence manufactured risk takes over. Even events previously held to be natural disasters, such as floods and famine, are now held to be avoidable consequences of human activities that must be risk-managed (Lupton 2011). As a result, society's governing institutions and expert bodies need to become ever more collectively self-aware of their role in the creation and management of risk (Beck and Beck-Gernsheim 2002). For the individual, meanwhile, uncertainties now litter their pathway through life to such an extent that it appears to be loaded with real and potential risks. So they must seek out and engage with a seemingly ever-growing number of information resources, provided by a myriad of sources, as they navigate through their world. In the risk society, '[we] find more and more guidebooks and practical manuals to do with health, diet, appearance, exercise, lovemaking and many other things' (Giddens 1991: 218).

Importantly, risk theorists such as Giddens and Beck talk about how we can see that since the 1960s and 1970s a growing cultural and political discourse of rights and responsibilities has been emerging, which seeks to regulate the individual while also arguing for the need for greater personal freedom. This leads us to a key feature of high modernity, which is arguably central to the study of contemporary developments in medical self-regulation. Namely, that within the risk society, a sense of growing (perhaps even mutual) distrust characterises the relationship between the public and experts (Giddens 1999). Yet at the same time, a pervasive and seemingly increasingly necessary reliance on an ever-growing number of experts appears to be a key feature of the individual's personal experience of everyday life (Mythen 2004).

Interestingly, it is argued that this established the conditions for the public to challenge elitism and expert forms of knowledge

(Chamberlain 2012). For under such changing social conditions, expert authority can no longer simply stand on the traditional basis of position and status – not least because an individual's growing need to manage risk and to problem-solve their everyday life, to make choices about who they are and what they should do, means that personal access to the technical and expert knowledge of the elite becomes more urgent than ever. The development of mass information-sharing tools, such as the mobile phone, the personal computer and the internet, mean that knowledge and expertise are no longer the sole preserve of those elite few who have undergone specialist training. As Giddens (1991) notes:

> technical knowledge is continually re-appropriated by lay agents … Modern life is a complex affair and there are many 'filter back' processes whereby technical knowledge, in one shape or another, is re-appropriated by lay persons and routinely applied in the course of their day-today activities … Processes of re-appropriation relate to all aspects of social life – for example, medical treatments, child rearing or sexual pleasure. (Giddens 1991: 144-6)

Governing medicine in the risk society

Osborne (1993) discusses how, since the re-emergence of liberalism, there has been a gradual reformulation of healthcare policy and practice, so that 'the field of medicine' is, to a greater degree than ever before, simultaneously both governed and self-governing. A key part of this process is the subjection of the activities of medical practitioners to an additional layer of management and new formal calculative regimes, such as performance indicators, competency frameworks and indicative budget targets. As Chapter One and Chapter Two discussed, this process began with the 1979 Conservative government, which possessed a firm neoliberal commitment to 'rolling back the state' and introducing free market philosophies within the public and private spheres (Rose 2000).

Thatcherism emphasised the entrepreneurial individual, endowed with freedom and autonomy and a self-reliant ability to care for herself, driven by the desire to optimise the worth of her own existence (Power 2007). For example, the Conservative home secretary Douglas Hurd stated in 1989 that 'the idea of active citizenship is a necessary complement to that of the enterprise culture' (quoted in Barnett 1991: 9). A new form of citizenship was being promoted by the changing conditions caused by the re-emergence of liberalism and having a direct effect on medical governance. Indeed, reviewing NHS reform during the mid-1990s, Johnson (1994) noted that:

> government-initiated change has, in recent reforms, been securely linked with the political commitment to the 'sovereign consumer'. In the case of reform in the National Health Service, this translates ... [to a] stress on prevention, the obligation to care for the self by adopting a healthy lifestyle, the commitment – shared with the new GP – to community care. (Johnson 1994: 149)

This state of affairs did not end with the election of 'New Labour' in 1997, or the Conservative–Liberal Democrat Coalition government in 2010. Indeed, over the last four decades changes in how expertise operates and is regulated, are arguably directed towards the object of good governance – the population in general and the individual subject-citizen in particular – as much as they are experts themselves (Rose 2000). Changes in how good citizenship is practised are bound up with shifts in the conditions under which good governance operates. In terms of Berlin's (1969) famous dichotomy of 'positive' and 'negative' liberty, although liberal mentalities of rule may appear at first to promote 'negative liberty' (that is, the personal freedom of the individual subject to decide who they are and discover what they want to be), in reality they promote 'positive liberty' (that is, a view of who and what a citizen-subject is and should be). As a result, there is an inherent tension between the key parties locked within the governing systems of control within Western democracies – governing social and political elites and the masses (Power 2007). The next section focuses on the consequences of this in the context of the media representation of instances of medical malpractice and criminality.

Doctors, patients and the media

Under the conditions of the risk society there is a tension between experts and citizens, between those in power and those who are not, and this can perhaps most clearly be seen in relation to modern technological advancements, particularly in relation to modern medicine and the provision and regulation of medical treatment and care (Chamberlain 2012). It can certainly be seen in the high-profile medical malpractice events outlined in previous chapters, including for example the subsequent formal governmental investigation of the Shipman case. It can also be seen in the fact that medical revalidation, as Chapter Two outlined, has not been greeted with enthusiasm by all members of the medical profession. As was noted, beliefs about the value of revalidation within the medical profession are certainly mixed: one study found that 15% of doctors thought that it would be of great value to the profession, 44% thought it would be of some value, 31% thought it would be of little value and 11% thought that it would be of no value (National Centre for Social Research 2014: 2).

Doctors' views of the value of revalidation for ensuring patient safety in this research were very similar: 12% of doctors thought that revalidation would be of great value to ensure patient safety, 39% thought it would be of some value, 34% thought it would be of little value and 15% thought that revalidation would be of no value to ensure patient safety. Only 12% of both men and women thought that revalidation would be of great value for patient safety (National Centre for Social Research 2014: 26). Similarly, as was also noted in Chapter Two, research by the King's Fund (2014: 1) found 'cynicism about the overarching purpose of assuring the public of doctors' fitness to practise'.

It is undoubtedly the case that revalidation has divided medical opinion in regard to the question of its utility as a developmental and quality assurance tool that benefits both the profession and the public. In no small part this is due to the fact that the media reporting of instances of medical underperformance is frequently seen as being unfairly skewed in favour of headline salaciousness rather than balanced informed opinion, by both 'rank and file' members of the profession and elite medical associations. This is particularly the case in the media reporting of alleged instances of medical malpractice where a doctor is unable to correct any inaccuracy or distortion, either prior to or after publication, without breaching client confidentiality (Williams et al 2014). With the result, as the GMC (2011: 1) notes, that: 'disputes between patients and doctors conducted in the media … may undermine public confidence in the profession'.

The GMC is increasingly operating in a multimedia age, which incorporates both traditional forms of globalised media (the 24-hour news media and the internet) and new forms of social media (such as Twitter, Facebook and WhatsApp), and it is undoubtedly the case that this is affecting – and will continue to affect – both the delivery of NHS services and the regulation of the healthcare professions. For example, in a 2012 report the Public Services Ombudsman for Wales (PSOW, 2012: 2) noted: 'I also believe that people are now more inclined to complain about poor service in the NHS than was previously the case and it is notable that almost half of health complaints are about clinical treatment in hospital'.

Freedom of speech and freedom of the press are essential elements of any advanced liberal democracy. There is a case to be made for the view that without growing media questioning of entrenched medical privilege and power from the 1970s onwards, the relatives of victims of medical malpractice and acts of criminality by doctors would not have received the justice they deserved (Chamberlain 2012). Nevertheless, it can equally be argued that it is important that the media does not engage in 'doctor-bashing' for its own sake. It has been noted that there is a clear tendency within the British media to imply that the GMC is ineffective, incompetent or still biased towards doctors (MacRae and Levy 2012, Robinson 2012). This situation will undoubtedly have an impact for better and worse on how both the GMC and political elites view medical regulation and respond to complaints. Indeed, McGivern and Fischer (2012: 291), in their report of interviews with people involved with or affected by regulatory transparency, quoted a medical member of the GMC saying: "if you're a doctor who's been criticised in the press … the GMC are very unlikely to find for you. It's definitely trial by media."

Perhaps the key question to ask here is: What is the impact of this situation on doctors and the regulation of medical expertise? Certainly, as Chapter Three discussed, it is important that current reforms to the fitness to practise tribunal process (proposed by the Law Commission), which appear to be primarily driven by matters of economic efficiency and practical expediency, do not become overly concerned with 'punishment for punishment's sake' as a key consequence of a risk-averse drive towards increased medical accountability and institutional transparency, in no small part due to the negative media coverage of high-profile cases such as Alder Hey, Bristol and Stafford (Case 2011). Similarly, as Chapter Two outlined, it is important that evaluation of the implementation of medical revalidation and its impact on improving clinical practice does not become overly focused on detecting problems and punishing individual doctors, but rather on how data sources and potential and actual risks are detected and managed at a systematic level to better support the developmental needs of doctors. The rest of this chapter will consider in detail whether the regulatory reforms outlined in previous chapters are indeed indicative of an overarching reform agenda that has become overly concerned with punishment.

Defensive medicine: is the process becoming the punishment?

As a result of externally and internally generated reform, medicine's training programmes, disciplinary mechanisms and regulatory inspection regimes all now possess clear standards that can be operationalised into performance outcomes against which the fitness to practise of members of the profession can be regularly checked in an apparently open, transparent and accountable manner (Chamberlain 2012). One consequence of this state of affairs has been the emergence of defensive medical practice as a seemingly legitimate – but nevertheless ultimately self-defeating – coping strategy (Allsop 2006). Defensive medicine occurs when diagnostic or therapeutic measures are used by a doctor as protection against possible accusations of negligence or underperformance, rather than because their patient really needs them (Summerton 1995, Studdert et al 2005). Studies show that doctors are increasingly engaging in defensive medicine as a result of a rise in healthcare managerialism, an increase in patient complaints and greater emphasis being placed on patient choice (Nettleton 2006, Gigerenzer 2014).

The emergence of defence medicine highlights that many 'rank and file' doctors feel pressured by the increased surveillance they are being placed under – from patients, the media, NHS clinical governance systems and their peers. Defensive decision making occurs in the healthcare arena because doctors are pursuing options that protect them in case something goes wrong, not because they are the most efficient and effective way of ensuring their patients' best interest. But what exactly are they afraid of? Could it be that they perceive the complaint-handling process not just to be inherently biased against them, but also stigmatising and damaging to their career, even in instances when it is recognised as being unfounded?

An apposite study here is Malcolm Feeley's (1979) sociolegal study *The Process is the Punishment*. On its publication, Feeley's empirical study of law in action in the lower criminal courts of New Haven, Connecticut, rapidly became an international classic of sociolegal research (Earle 2008). Feeley highlighted that in some instances, due process procedural safeguards designed to preserve the right to trial by jury were undermined by the severity of pre-trial punishments (for example, the economic costs associated with paying bail bondsmen or retaining counsel). He noted that the pre-trial process often served the function of punishing the defendant, with court actors other than the judge and jury, such as bail bondsmen, possessing a key role in the administration of punishment, as they often incentivised the defendant to plead guilty. One of the key reasons why this was the case, as Feeley outlined, was the fact that becoming engaged in the system itself generates a cost to defendants not only directly, but indirectly as well:

> For every defendant sentenced to a jail term of any length, there are likely to be several others who were released from jail only after and because they pleaded guilty. For each dollar paid out in fines, a defendant is likely to have spent four or five dollars for a bondsman and an attorney. For each dollar they lose in fines, working defendants likely lose several more from docked wages. For every defendant who has lost his job because of a conviction, there are probably five more who have lost their jobs as a result of simply having missed work in order to appear in court. ... When we view criminal sanctioning from this broader, functional perspective, the locus of court-imposed sanctioning shifts dramatically away from adjudication, plea bargaining, and sentencing to the earlier pre-trial stages. In essence, the process itself is the punishment. (Feeley 1979: 30–1)

In the context of the hearing of fitness to practise cases, there is a growing body of research indicating that pre-hearing investigative measures are traumatising doctors who suffer from health-related problems in particular, and in some instances this is leading them to agree to high-impact sanctions, namely suspension or erasure from the medical register, *before* they attend an FPP hearing, with the hearing subsequently becoming a 'rubber stamp' exercise (Moberly 2014). Moreover, the fact that 96 doctors have died while facing a fitness to practise investigation since 2004 suggests that there are legitimate questions in regard to the overly punitive nature of the process. While it is not possible to provide a breakdown of the figures in terms of deaths by suicide, the GMC has nonetheless launched a review of the number of suicides of doctors facing fitness to practise hearings, which will be published in 2015 (GMC 2014). For the moment it is important to highlight that McGivern and Fischer (2012: 291) note that one of their research participants (a general practitioner) told them about a colleague who "got a letter from the GMC one morning ... On the day she needed to attend, she hung herself." Samanta and Samanta (2004: 212) quote a study of 105 doctors who had been suspended through one or other disciplinary routes: 'One third required treatment for medical problems directly attributable to the suspension, one third had sought psychiatric help and about half declared that a family member, usually the spouse, have suffered ill health as a consequence'.

Certainly, these issues lend weight to the position (often held by 'rank and file' practitioners) that the GMC appears to operate a default assumption that complainants are correct and honest in their representations. Regardless of the arguments for and against the truth of this proposition, the growing evidence of the negative effects of the complaints process on doctors' health lends weight to the view that it is the *process* itself which is of principal importance in determining whether procedural fairness has been achieved and appropriate punishment delivered, and not the individual outcome of a given procedure (Galligan 1996). In addition, procedural justice scholars have observed that an individual's experience of the process strongly influences the *perceived* fairness of the substantive result of a legal process (Tyler 1988, Solum 2004).

As a result, reformers ought not to identify a numerical increase in enquiries about doctors being investigated and called to account for their actions, as a key measure from which to judge their success or otherwise in reforming medical regulation. Instead, greater attention should be paid to examining whether doctors, patients and their respective legal representatives report greater satisfaction with the case hearing process, even when the hearing outcome does not find in their favour. Such an endeavour would be useful in generating better understanding of conceptions of fair treatment, impartiality and equity, within the domain of fitness to practise hearings.

Research suggests that both patients and medical practitioners have previously reported high levels of dissatisfaction with how the GMC responds to complaints (National Centre for Social Research 2014). Given the naturally competing interests of both parties, this is somewhat to be expected. However, the director of the London-based

Practitioner Health Programme, which has supported many doctors going through GMC investigations, has recently commented that the GMC is traumatising doctors and may be harming patients (Moberly 2014). This is clearly an unacceptable state of affairs. The fitness to practise hearing is the only mechanism for providing fairness in procedure, and for achieving a balance between the competing interests of parties to ensure greater satisfaction with the tribunal process. It must, therefore, remain a strategic priority for government when it intervenes in medical regulation with reforming intentions, to ensure that the legislative system it enacts is equitable and fit for purpose.

Conclusion

Given these considerations, it is imperative that critical observers continue to pay close critical attention to the evolving nature of legislative developments pertaining to the regulation of medical practitioners, particularly in relation to the consequences of reform for the independence of the fitness to practise tribunal process, to ensure procedural fairness. The Law Commission recommendation that the Medical Practitioners Tribunal Service become an autonomous structure within the organisation of the GMC, as outlined in Chapter Three, seeks to balance state concerns over cost, with a legitimate professional concern with maintaining a necessary element of strong discretion within professional regulatory frameworks. Only time will tell if this is indeed a viable alternative to the creation of a separate body undertaking FPP hearing and adjudication. Whatever happens next in the development of the GMC and how it responds to cases which raise concern about a doctor's fitness to practise, the shift towards risk-averse forms of professional accountability must not sacrifice due process in the name of political pragmatic exigency.

At the beginning of this book it was noted that the introduction of medical revalidation and reforms to the hearing of fitness to practise cases signifies the end of the idea that doctors can be trusted to be left alone to manage their own affairs. In tracing the reforms made over the last four decades, it has been argued that a new regulatory bargain has been struck between the profession and the public, and furthermore, that the use of risk-based quality assurance frameworks has enhanced the ability of the regulatory systems in place to more readily identify and deal with instances of medical underperformance, malpractice and criminality.

Only time will tell what the full impact of the reforming agenda will be. But one thing is certain: the balance of power and control has not shifted away from doctors and towards patients. Rather it is shifting towards specialist groups, some of whom operate inside the medical profession and some of whom operate outside it. Although they may disagree on many things, nevertheless they share the belief that risk-averse systems of surveillance and control are the best way forward in ensuring rigour, transparency and accountability in medical regulation. Whether or not this does indeed lead to improved service provision and protection for the public, is a question that only time can answer.

References

Allsop, J (2006) Regaining Trust in Medicine: Professional and State Strategies, *Current Sociology*, 54, 4: 621–36

Barnett, M (1991) *The Politics of Truth* (Cambridge: Polity Press)

Beck, U (1992) *Risk Society: Towards a New Modernity* (London: Sage Publications)

Beck, U and Beck-Gernsheim, E (2002) *Individualization: Institutionalized Individualism and its Social and Political Consequences* (London: Sage Publications)

Berlin, I (1969) Two Concepts of Liberty, in Berlin, I (2002) *Four Essays on Liberty* (Oxford: Oxford University Press)

Case, P (2011) Putting Public Confidence First: Doctors, Precautionary Suspension and the General Medical Council, *Medical Law Review*, 19: 339–71

Chamberlain, J M (2012) *The Sociology of Medical Regulation: An Introduction* (London: Springer)

Dent, M, Chandler, M and Barry, J (2004) *Questioning the New Public Management* (Aldershot: Ashgate)

Earle, J (2008) The Process is the Punishment: Thirty Years Later, *Law and Social Inquiry*, 33: 737-40

Feeley, M (1979) *The Process is the Punishment: Handling Cases in a Lower Criminal Court* (CT: Russell Sage Foundation)

Galligan, D J (1996) *Due Process and Fair Procedures* (Oxford: Clarendon Press)

General Medical Council (GMC) (2011) *Record Number of Complaints and Disciplinary Hearings Against Doctors*, Press Release, 24 October 2011 (London: GMC)

GMC (2014) *Chief Executive's Report* (London: GMC)

Giddens, A (1990) *The Consequences of Modernity* (Cambridge: Polity Press)

Giddens, A (1991) *Modernity and Self-Identity: Self and Society in Late Modernity* (Cambridge: Policy Press)

Giddens, A (1999) Risk and Responsibility, *Modern Law Review*, 62, 1: 1–10

Gigerenzer, G (2014) *Risk Savvy: How to Make Good Decisions* (NY: Viking)

Glynne, J and Gomez, D (2005) *Fitness to Practice: Health Care Regulatory Law, Principle, and Process* (London: Thomson, Sweet and Maxwell)

Havighurst, C C (1991) Practice Guidelines as Legal Standards Governing Physician Liability, *Law and Contemporary Problems*, 54: 87-8

Hood, C (2002) The Risk Game and the Blame Game, *Government and Opposition*, 37: 15-37

Hutter, B and Power, M (2005) *Organisational Encounters with Risk* (Cambridge: Cambridge University Press)

Johnson, T J (1994) Expertise and The State, in Gane, M and Johnson, T J (eds) *Foucault's New Domains* (London: Routledge)

Kings Fund (2014) *Revalidation: From Compliance to Commitment* London: Kings Fund

Lupton D (2011) *Risk* London: Routledge

MacRae, F and Levy, A (2012) Three-quarters of doctors who are struck off in Britain are trained abroad, *Mail Online*, 31 December 2012

McGivern, G and Fischer, M (2012) Reactivity and Reactions to Regulatory Transparency in Medicine, Psychotherapy and Counselling, *Social Science and Medicine*, 74: 289-96

Moberly, T (2014) GMC is Traumatising Unwell Doctors and May Be Undermining Patient Safety, *BMJ Careers*, 20: 10-11

Mythen, G (2004) *Ulrich Beck: A Critical Introduction to the Risk Society* (London: Pluto)

National Centre for Social Research (2014) *Fairness and the GMC: Doctors' Views* (London: NCSR)

Nettleton, S (2006) *The Sociology of Health and Illness* (Bristol: Policy Press)

Osborne, T (1993) On Liberalism, Neo-Liberalism and the Liberal Profession of Medicine, *Economy and Society*, 22, 3: 345-56

Power, M (2007) *Organised Uncertainty: Designing a World of Risk Management* (Oxford: Oxford University Press)

Public Services Ombudsman for Wales (PSOW) (2012) *Annual Report 2011-2012* (Cardiff: PSOW)

Robinson, M (2012) 'A danger to patients': Twice suspended doctor who prescribed wrong drugs and did unauthorised operations back at work, *Daily Mail*, 11 April 2012

Rose, N. (2000) *Powers of Freedom: Reframing Political Thought* (Cambridge: Cambridge University Press)

Samanta, A and Samanta, J (2004) Regulation of the Medical Profession: Fantasy, Reality and Legality, *Journal Royal Society Medicine*, 97: 211-18

Scrivens, E (2007) The Future of Regulation and Governance, *Journal of the Royal Society for the Promotion of Health*, 127: 72-7

Solum, L B (2004) Procedural Justice, *Southern California Law Review*, 78: 181-221

Studdert, D M, Mello, M M, Sage, W M, DesRoches, C M, Peugh, J, Zapert, K and Brennan, T A (2005) Defensive Medicine Among High-risk Specialist Physicians in a Volatile Malpractice Environment, *Journal of American Medical Association*, 293: 2609-17

Summerton, N (1995) Positive and Negative Factors in Defensive Medicine: A Questionnaire Study of General Practitioners, *BMJ*, 310: 27-8

Tyler, T (1988) What is Procedural Justice?, *Law and Society Review*, 22: 103-35

Waring, J and Dixon-Woods, M (2010) Modernising Medical Regulation: Where Are We Now?, *Journal of Health Organisation and Management*, 24: 540-55

Williams, H, Lees, C and Boyd, M (2014) *The General Medical Council: Fit to Practice?* (London: CIVITAS)

NOTES

[1]   The law requires all private and NHS doctors who treat patients in the United Kingdom be registered with the GMC and issued with a license to practice. This list is commonly referred to as 'the medical register', with each doctor having their own individual 'GMC number' for identification purposes. For pragmatic reasons, the register includes two important subgroups - the specialist register (a list of all consultant level doctors which was first introduced in 1997) and the general practice register (a list of all doctors in general practice which was first introduced in 2001)

[2]   (1957) *Bolam* v *Friem Hospital Management Committee*, 1 WLR 582, 121.

[3]   (1957) *Bolam* v *Friem Hospital Management Committee*, 1 WLR 582, 121.

[4]   (1957) *Bolam* v *Friem Hospital Management Committee*, 1 WLR, 587.

[5]   (1985) *Sidaxazy* v *Board of Governors of the Bethlem Royal Hospital and the Maudsley Hospital*, 1 AC 871, 881.

[6]   (1985) *Sidaxazy* v *Board of Governors of the Bethlem Royal Hospital and the Maudsley Hospital*, 1 AC 871, 881.

[7]   (1985) *Sidaxazy* v *Board of Governors of the Bethlem Royal Hospital and the Maudsley Hospital*, 1 AC 871, 609.

[8]   As listed in the Chapter Three references: GMC 2000; GMC 2001; GMC 2002; GMC 2003; GMC 2004b; GMC 2005; GMC 2006; GMC 2007; GMC 2008; GMC 2009; GMC 2010; GMC 2011a; GMC 2012; GMC 2013b.

THE GOOD MEDICAL PRACTICE FRAMEWORK FOR APPRAISAL AND REVALIDATION

The GMP framework for appraisal and revalidation (General Medical Council 2014) sets out four broad domain areas which should be covered in a doctor's appraisal and on which the recommendations to revalidate doctors should be based. As Chapter Two discusses, these domains also set the basis from which revalidation can be evaluated as a quality assurance tool.

Domain 1 – Knowledge, skills and performance

1.1 Maintain your professional performance

- Maintain knowledge of the law and other regulation relevant to your work
- Keep knowledge and skills about your current work up to date
- Participate in professional development and educational activities
- Take part in and respond constructively to the outcome of systematic quality improvement activities (eg audit), appraisals and performance reviews

1.2 Apply knowledge and experience to practise

- Recognise and work within the limits of your competence
- If you work in research, follow appropriate national research governance guidelines
- If you are a teacher/trainer, apply the skills, attitudes and practice of a competent teacher/trainer
- If you are a manager, work effectively as a manager
- Support patients in caring for themselves
- If you are in a clinical role:
  - Adequately assess the patient's conditions
  - Provide or arrange advice, investigations or treatment where necessary
  - Prescribe drugs or treatment, including repeat prescriptions, safely and appropriately
  - Provide effective treatments based on the best available evidence
  - Take steps to alleviate pain and distress whether or not a cure may be possible
  - Consult colleagues, or refer patients to colleagues, when this is in the patient's best interests

1.3 Ensure that all documentation (including clinical records) formally recording your work is clear, accurate and legible

- Make and/or review records at the same time as the events are documented or as soon as possible afterwards
- Ensure that any documentation that records your findings, decisions, information given to patients, drugs prescribed and other information or treatment is up to date and accurate
- Implement and comply with systems to protect patient confidentiality

Domain 2 – Safety and quality

2.1 Contribute to and comply with systems to protect patients

- Take part in systems of quality assurance and quality improvement
- Comply with risk management and clinical governance procedures
- Cooperate with legitimate requests for information from organisations monitoring public health
- Provide information for confidential inquiries, significant event reporting
- Make sure that all staff for whose performance you are responsible, including locums and students, are properly supervised
- Report suspected adverse reactions
- Ensure arrangements are made for the continuing care of the patient where necessary
- Ensure systems are in place for colleagues to raise concerns about risks to patients

2.2 Respond to risks to safety

- Report risks in the healthcare environment to your employing or contracting bodies
- Safeguard and protect the health and well-being of vulnerable people, including children and the elderly and those with learning disabilities
- Take action where there is evidence that a colleague's conduct, performance or health may be putting patients at risk
- Respond promptly to risks posed by patients
- Follow infection control procedures and regulations

2.3 Protect patients and colleagues from any risk posed by your health

- Make arrangements for accessing independent medical advice when necessary

- Be immunised against common serious communicable diseases where vaccines are available

Domain 3 – Communication, partnership and teamwork

3.1 Communicate effectively

- Listen to patients and respect their views about their health
- Give patients the information they need in order to make decisions about their care in a way they can understand
- Respond to patients' questions
- Keep patients informed about the progress of their care
- Explain to patients when something has gone wrong
- Treat those close to the patient considerately
- Communicate effectively with colleagues within and outside the team
- Encourage colleagues to contribute to discussions and to communicate effectively with each other
- Pass on information to colleagues involved in, or taking over, your patients' care

3.2 Work constructively with colleagues and delegate effectively

- Treat colleagues fairly and with respect
- Support colleagues who have problems with their performance, conduct or health
- Act as a positive role model for colleagues
- Ensure colleagues to whom you delegate have appropriate qualifications and experience
- Provide effective leadership as appropriate to their role

3.3 Establish and maintain partnerships with patients

- Encourage patients to take an interest in their health and to take action to improve and maintain it

- Be satisfied that you have consent or other valid authority before you undertake any examination or investigation, provide treatment or involve patients in teaching or research

Domain 4 – Maintaining trust

4.1 Show respect for patients

- Implement and comply with systems to protect patient confidentiality
- Be polite, considerate and honest and respect patients' dignity and privacy
- Treat each patient fairly and as an individual
- If you undertake research, respect the rights of patients participating in the research

4.2 Treat patients and colleagues fairly and without discrimination

- Be honest and objective when appraising or assessing colleagues and when writing references
- Respond promptly and fully to complaints
- Provide care on the basis of the patient's needs and the likely effect of treatment

4.3 Act with honesty and integrity

- Ensure you have adequate indemnity or insurance cover for your practice
- Be honest in financial and commercial dealings
- Ensure any published information about your services is factual and verifiable
- Be honest in any formal statement or report, whether written or oral, making clear the limits of your knowledge or competence
- Inform patients about any fees and charges before starting treatment

- If you undertake research, obtain appropriate ethical approval and honestly report results

INDEX

A

adjudication stage, complaint handling, 64
adjudicators, independent, 37
Annual Appraisals, 35
appeals to complaints, 65
appraisal, introduction of, 29–30
audits *see* medical audits
autonomy of doctors, 3

B

Bolam test, 12, 81
Bolam v Friem Hospital Management Committee, 12
Bolitho gloss, 12–13, 81
Bolitho v City and Hackney Health Authority, 12–13
Bristol Royal Infirmary, 6–7
British Medical Association (BMA), 27

C

Case Quality Commission, 62
Catto, Graeme, 34–35
clinical freedom, 10–11
clinical performance, self-surveillance, 45
club governance models, 3–4
communication, *The Good Medical Practice Framework for Appraisal and Revalidation* (GMC 2014), 102–103
complaints
 appeals to, 65
 as marker of patient trust, 15
 Professional Standards Authority, 8–9
  stages of, 63–64
  see also GMC adjudication processes
Conservative government (1979), 25
continuing professional development (CPD), 30
Council for Healthcare Regulatory Excellence (CHRE) *see* Professional Standards Authority (PSA)
Court of Session, 65
CPD (continuing professional development), 30
criminal convictions, 63–64

D

defensive medicine, 88–92
deferral requests, 40, 52
Dhasmana, Janardan, 6–7
disengagement, revalidation, 49
Donaldson, Liam, 37
Duties of a Doctor (GMC 1995), 31–32

E

education continuation, 26–29
 monitoring strategies, 27
electronic portfolios, 42–43
end-user cynicism, revalidation, 49
enthusiasts, performance appraisal, 47
evidence-based medicine, 28
external risk, 82–83

F

Feeley, Malcolm, 89–90
fitness to practise cases, Professional Standards Authority, 8–9
fitness to practise panels (FPP), 2, 59–60, 72–76, 80

changes to, 37
complaints handling, 63–65
as marker of trust, 15
outcomes, 64–65, 70, 71t, 72
pre-meeting sanctions, 90–91
referrals to, 65
reform of, 74
  see also Medical Practitioners
  Tribunal Service (MPTS)
formal social control, 11–12
Foucauldian interpretation,
  revalidation, 42–45
framework, The Good Medical
  Practice Framework for Appraisal and
  Revalidation (GMC 2014), 102–103
freedom of speech, 87–88
freedom of the press, 87–88

G

GMC (General Medical Council)
  bias to doctors, 80
  board members, 5, 8
  changes in, 18, 36, 60, 61, 79–80
  criticisms of, 80
  establishment, 4
  membership changes, 34
  non-medical lay membership, 37
GMC adjudication processes, 62–72
  assumed correctness of complaints,
    91
  enquiry number, 66–68, 67t
  investigatory and adjudicatory role
    separation, 75
  investigatory stage outcome, 69–70,
    69t
  source of enquiry, 67–68, 68t
  see also complaints; Medical
    Practitioners Tribunal Service
    (MPTS)
GMC affiliate see responsible officer
  (RO)
good citizenship, 85
Good Medical Practice (GMC 2013a),
  29–30, 31–32, 39, 63
The Good Medical Practice Framework
  for Appraisal and Revalidation (GMC
  2014), 39, 99–104

communication, partnership and
  teamwork, 102–103
knowledge, skills and performance,
  99–100
safety and quality, 101–102
trust maintenance, 103–104
governing of medicine, 84–86
the Griffiths Report, 25
Griffiths, Roy, 25

H

Health and Social Care Act (2008), 3,
  6–10, 37–38, 60, 72–73
Health and Social Care Act (2012), 3
High Court, 65, 74
history of regulation, 1–21
Hospital Consultants and Specialists
  Committee (HCSC), 33
hospital management, 24–26
Hurd, Douglas, 85

I

independent adjudicators, 37
informal social control, 11–12
information panopticon, 44
interim orders panel, 64
investigation stage
  complaint handling, 63–64
  outcomes, 69–70, 69t, 70t
Irvine, Donald, 31

J

Jeffreys, Margot, 31

K

Kennedy, Ian, 6–7, 26
knowledge, The Good Medical
  Practice Framework for Appraisal and
  Revalidation (GMC 2014), 99–100

L

Law Commission Review, 72–76, 92
local disciplinary procedures, 52
local implementation of revalidation,
  38–42

M

manufactured risk, 82–83
media, 86–88
Medical Act (1858), 3, 4–6

Medical Act (1983), 59, 63
Medical (Professional Performance)
    Act 1995, 31
medical audits, 28
 introduction of, 16
Medical Education (Southgate 2001),
    32
medical expertise, 10–12
medical game-playing, 16–17
 performance appraisal, 46
medical malpractice cases on TV, 26
Medical Practitioners Tribunal
    Service (MPTS), 2, 59–78
 autonomy recommendations, 92
 complaint handling, 62–65
 establishment of, 74
 independence of, 75
 medical fitness to practise, 62–65
 see also fitness to practise panels
    (FPP); GMC adjudication processes
Medical Profession (Responsible
    Officers) Regulations 2010/2013,
    38
medical register, 4, 59
 removal from, 30
medical regulation
 history of, 1–21
 necessity for, 9–10
 risk-based regulation, 14–17
 self-regulation *see* self-regulation
meso-regulators, 9
Mid-Staffordshire NHS Trust, 60–61
minimalists, performance appraisal, 47

N

National Centre for Social Research,
    49
National Clinical Assessment Service,
    62
National Health Service (NHS)
 appraisals, 38, 45
 criticism, 88
 establishment, 4, 24–25
 reforms, 25–26, 33, 85
National Health Service Reform and
    Health Care Professions Act 2002,
    65, 74–75
negative liberty, 85

New Public Management, 80–81
NHS England, 38
NHS Management Inquiry (1983), 25
The NHS Plan (2000), 29
non-compliers, performance
    appraisal, 46–47
non-engagement, 40–41
non-medical input in revalidation, 41

O

Office of Healthy Professions
    Adjudication (OHPA), 73
official professional discretion, 11

P

paper-based portfolios, 42–43
paperwork compliance, 47–48
Parliamentary and Health Service
    Ombudsman, 62
partnership, *The Good Medical
    Practice Framework for Appraisal and
    Revalidation* (GMC 2014), 102–103
The Patient's Charter (DOH 1991), 25
performance, *The Good Medical
    Practice Framework for Appraisal and
    Revalidation* (GMC 2014), 99–100
performance appraisal
 appraisal of, 45–48
 paperwork compliance, 47–48
portfolio-based performance appraisal,
    42–43, 49–50
positive liberty, 85
positive recommendations, 40
The Process is the Punishment (Feeley),
    89–90
professional discretion, 10–12, 16–17
 types of, 11
Professional Standards Authority
    (PSA), 8–9
 fitness to practise panels decision
    review, 65
 necessity for, 73–74
protectionism, 36
Public Appointments Committee,
    8, 37
public expenditure reduction, 25
Public Services Ombudsman for
    Wales (PSOW 2012:2), 87

Q

quality, *The Good Medical Practice Framework for Appraisal and Revalidation* (GMC 2014), 101–102

R

realistic prospect test, 61–62
recertification of specialists, 38
Reid, John, 37
relicensing, 38
responsible officer (RO), 38–41
  qualifications, 39
  recommendations to GMC, 40–41, 52
  responsibilities, 39
Revalidating Doctors: Ensuring Standards, Securing the Future (GMC 2000), 24
revalidation, 2, 17, 23–58
  appraisal of, 50–51
  doctors' views on, 86
  effect on doctors' behaviour, 49
  Foucauldian interpretation, 42–45
  implementation, 60
  introduction of, 9–10, 30–32
  local implementation, 38–42
  non-medical input, 41
  perceived value, 48–50
  portfolio-based performance appraisal, 42–43
  self-identified learning goals, 45
  supporting information, 43
Revalidation Support Team, 48–49
Revalidation: What You Need to Do (GMC 2013b), 39
risk-based regulation, 14–17
risk society, 81–84
  governing medicine, 84–86
Roylace, John, 6–7

S

Sadaxazy v Board of Governors of the Bethlem Royal Hospital and the Maudsley Hospital, 12
safety, *The Good Medical Practice Framework for Appraisal and Revalidation* (GMC 2014), 101–102

self-identified learning goals, revalidation, 45
self-regulation, 10–11
  changes to, 41–42
service orientation, 23–24
Shipman, Harold, 7–8, 24, 34
Siebel computer system, 14–15
skills, *The Good Medical Practice Framework for Appraisal and Revalidation* (GMC 2014), 99–100
Smith, Janet, 8, 34–35
Smith, Richard, 30
social control, 11–12
specialist medicine, development of, 5–6
specialist recertification, 38
Stacey, Margaret, 6, 31
strong professional discretion, 11
Supporting Doctors, Protecting Patients (DOH 1999), 33
supporting information, revalidation, 43

T

television programmes, medical malpractice cases, 26

U

UMbRELLA (Uk Medical Revalidation Evaluation coLLaboration), 53
'The Unmasking of Medicine' (Kennedy 1983), 26

W

weak professional discretion, 11
Wisheart, James, 6–7
Working for Patients (DOH 1989), 25

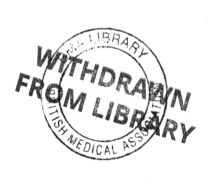